WHAT SOCIAL WORKERS NEED TO KNOW

Social work deals with the heavy end of human difficulties such as cruelty, self-destructiveness, and severe and enduring mental health problems. How do social workers make sense of the emotional difficulties which come with the realities of practice? Understanding our clients is the best way of dealing with complex situations and avoiding burnout and stress. The contributors to this book argue that psychoanalysis provides a theory of development and behaviour capable of formulating a realistic model for understanding emotional difficulties and disturbances in both clients and ourselves.

The chapters demonstrate a way of thinking for the practitioner that can be used in all situations. The book examines in detail some of the difficult and disturbing conversations that social workers have with clients of all ages. It provides a psycho-analytic framework for understanding circumstances which may be puzzling, stressful or frightening, and a theory whose value for many social work problems is well underpinned by research evidence.

Written by senior practitioners who are all still working in the front line, this book puts complex real life experiences into words, to help the social worker become a more effective practitioner.

Marion Bower is a freelance social worker and adult psychotherapist. She has worked in child and family mental health services for 34 years including 14 years at the Tavistock Clinic. She co-edited *The Emotional Needs of Young Children and Their Families* and edited *Psychoanalytic Theory for Social Work Practice*, both published by Routledge, and *Addictive States of Mind*.

Robin Solomon worked as a consultant social worker at the Tavistock Clinic where she held senior roles in both clinical work and teaching. She is a senior fellow of the Higher Education Academy and is a Trustee of the Centre for Social Work Practice. Robin is currently working as an independent consultant and visiting lecturer.

WHAT SOCIAL WORKERS NEED TO KNOW

A Psychoanalytic Approach

Edited by Marion Bower and Robin Solomon

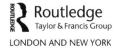

Routledge
Taylor & Francis Group

LONDON AND NEW YORK

First published 2018
by Routledge
2 Park Square, Milton Park, Abingdon, Oxon OX14 4RN

and by Routledge
711 Third Avenue, New York, NY 10017

Routledge is an imprint of the Taylor & Francis Group, an informa business

British Library Cataloguing in Publication Data
A catalogue record for this book is available from the British Library

Library of Congress Cataloging in Publication Data
Names: Bower, Marion, 1949- editor. | Solomon, Robin (Social worker), editor.
Title: What social workers need to know : a psychoanalytic approach / edited by Marion Bower and Robin Solomon.
Description: Abingdon, Oxon ; New York, NY : Routledge, 2017. | Includes bibliographical references and index.
Identifiers: LCCN 2017011070 | ISBN 9781138905634 (hardback) | ISBN 9781138905665 (pbk.) | ISBN 9781315695815 (ebook)
Subjects: LCSH: Social workers--Job stress--Great Britain. | Social service--Practice--Great Britain.
Classification: LCC HV40.8.G7 W43 2017 | DDC 361.301/9--dc23
LC record available at https://lccn.loc.gov/2017011070

ISBN: 978-1-138-90563-4 (hbk)
ISBN: 978-1-138-90566-5 (pbk)
ISBN: 978-1-315-69581-5 (ebk)

Typeset in Bembo
by Taylor & Francis Books

Printed and bound by CPI Group (UK) Ltd, Croydon, CR0 4YY

CONTENTS

FIGURES

CONTRIBUTORS

James Blewett is currently based in the Social Care Workforce Research Unit at King's College London, and is the research director and chair of the national research dissemination network, Making Research Count. He has previously worked at Royal Holloway, the Open University and Kingston University.

Sophie Boswell is a psychoanalytic psychotherapist working with children and adults. She qualified as a child psychotherapist at the Tavistock Centre in 2003, subsequently working and teaching in various settings including children's CAMHS community settings, children's centres, schools and nurseries. For several years she worked in a CAMHS team within Westminster's Looked After Children department. She was also a member of Westminster's Adoption and Permanency Panel, and a member of the NICE panel, producing guidelines on the *Wellbeing of Looked After Children* (2010). Sophie is the author of *Understanding Your Baby* (2003), part of the Tavistock's Understanding Your Child series. She currently works in private practice in London.

Susan Chantrell is a child and adolescent psychotherapist trained at the Tavistock Clinic, London. She previously worked in an NHS Child and Adolescent Mental Health Service and in the Tavistock Learning and Complex Disabilities Service.

Andrew Cooper is Professor of Social Work at the Tavistock Centre and University of East London. He is a registered social worker and psychoanalytic psychotherapist. He researches and writes extensively about relationship based and therapeutic social work practice, as well as the interplay between societal dynamics and organisational and practice milieus. With Julian Lousada he wrote *Borderline Welfare: Feeling and Fear of Feeling in Modern Welfare* (2005, Karnac) and a collection of his papers *Conjunctions: Between Social Work, Psychoanalysis and Society* will be published in 2017 in the Tavistock Clinic book series.

Lynne Cudmore originally trained as a social worker, working for seven years in a social services department in London. She then trained and worked for 26 years as a psychoanalytic psychotherapist for couple relationships at the Tavistock Centre for Couple Relationships. Her research interests there included the impact of infertility on the couple relationship and the impact of a child's death on the couple. She was the programme leader for the Professional Doctorate in Couple Psychoanalytic Psychotherapy. She trained as a child psychotherapist at the Tavistock Clinic and went on to work in the Infant Mental Health Team there. She later became a Consultant Child Psychotherapist in the Family Mental Health Team and founded the service for teenage parents at the Tavistock. For six years she worked in a CAMHS team based in the Looked After Children's team in Westminster Children's Services, and currently works as a Consultant Child Psychotherapist in the Perinatal Mental Health Team at Chelsea and Westminster Hospital.

Anna Harvey is a senior clinical lecturer in social work and social care. She has been a children and families social worker for 20 years and has 27 years' experience in the caring professions. She is an advanced practitioner and is an experienced expert witness in care proceedings. She has worked as a reflective practice supervisor for the past 10 years. She has a research interest in the emotional aspects of decision-making in child protection practice and has completed her professional doctorate in social care and emotional wellbeing.

Fiona Henderson is a clinical psychologist and psychoanalytic psychotherapist in the NHS. Formerly consultant adult psychotherapist in the Monroe Family Assessment Service of the Tavistock Clinic, she has worked with disturbed parents involved in care proceedings and has an interest in how personality difficulties affect parenting through the generations. Her doctorate was a study of psychoanalytic aspects of communication during social work home visits and she is involved in teaching and training in this area.

Narendra Keval is an adult and adolescent psychotherapist and consultant clinical psychologist. He worked as a specialist in psychoanalytic psychotherapy in a range of NHS settings with patients suffering from complex personality disorders. He is a visiting lecturer at the Tavistock Clinic, London, and a visiting speaker on psychoanalytic training programmes in Washington and New York. He is a member of the Tavistock Society of Psychotherapists and is currently in full-time private practice. His book *Racist States of Mind: Understanding the Perversion of Curiosity and Concern* was published recently with Karnac Books.

Charlotte Noyes is an independent social worker and reviewing officer. She is a registered social worker who has over 25 years' experience of working with children and families, mainly in the statutory sector within London. In 2016 she was awarded the Professional Doctorate in Social Work at the Tavistock Centre/University of East London.

Gill Rusbridger trained as a social worker, working initially in adult mental health and later with children and families in a paediatric department. She trained as an adult psychotherapist and is a Senior Member of the British Psychotherapy Foundation. She is the Trust Wide Head of Social Work and works and teaches in the Child, Young Adolescent and Family Directorate at the Tavistock and Portman NHS Foundation Trust. She has a private psychotherapy practice with adults, and is a Training Therapist for the Westminster Pastoral Foundation.

Joanne Stubley is a consultant psychiatrist in psychotherapy at the Tavistock Clinic. She leads the Tavistock Trauma Service, and has considerable experience of working with individuals, groups and organisations who have experienced trauma. She is actively involved in teaching and training in this field, with a particular interest in complex trauma. Dr Stubley is a member of the British Psychoanalytic Society, and is trained in Trauma Focused Cognitive Behavioural Therapy (tf-CBT) and Eye Movement Desensitisation and Reprocessing (EMDR).

ACKNOWLEDGEMENTS

Marion Bower

We are grateful to Routledge for putting up with our slow progress with the book. This has allowed it to grow organically, with chapters added as the need arose. Thanks also go to Karnac Books for permission to reprint Narendra Keval's chapter 'Psychoanalysis and the Psychotherapies – Institutional Cleansing'. A few minor modifications have been made to bring the political references up to date.

Our students at Royal Holloway, University of London and the Tavistock Clinic were the catalyst for new ideas. Marion Bower is very grateful to the student who said, during a lecture, 'is this psychoanalysis? We like it'.

Our contributors put up with requests for changes and, in some cases, impossible deadlines. We are grateful for their ideas. Not all of them are social workers, but they have worked in social work settings, and know the sort of issues social workers have to face.

Our thanks go to James Blewett at King's College London's 'Making Research Count'. He enabled us to try out some of our ideas on experienced social workers for continuing professional development seminars.

Special thanks go to our Assistant Editor, Bruno Bower. It is literally true that without him the book would not have happened. Steve Bower was supportive as always, and Jacob Bower gave good advice. Sid the cat did his bit.

Robin Solomon

I would like first to acknowledge my partner Mike Squires for his endless patience and knowing how important this was to me. To Marion, my co-editor who took me under her wing as a fledgling editor. A special thanks to Harry Venning whose cover illustration captured just what we wanted to convey – social work meets psychoanalysis – brilliantly!

Anita Colloms, if you ever come across this you were part of this journey, as was Joan DiBlasi my first supervisor and life-long friend. To Susan, because you have filled a gap. And to all of my patients, colleagues and students, who over many years have taught me the value of a psychoanalytic perspective. I hope this volume does you all justice.

I would like to dedicate the book to my parents, in whose minds I was lovingly held and who I have come to appreciate more through my encounters with psychoanalytic thinking. I regret that it did not make it to your coffee table in time.

1

INTRODUCTION

What social workers need to know

Marion Bower and Robin Solomon

This is a unique social work book. We are fortunate to have four chapters based on in-depth research, so we are able to talk about social work as it really is. Our other chapters describe new ways of thinking about key social work issues. Our authors demonstrate, using case material, how psychoanalytic theory can underpin effective interventions. Finally we suggest how some of these ideas can be integrated into social work training. A chapter by James Blewett describes the context of social work today.

We have not covered every aspect of social work. Our criteria for chapters are that they can increase the reader's understanding of human nature. We have also added an afterword to the end of each chapter to contribute further ideas on the topic. Not all our authors are social workers, although they have all worked with social work problems. We feel it is an opportunity for social workers to hear from psychologists, psychiatrists and child psychotherapists. The book is the equivalent of a multi-disciplinary team. This is a companion volume to *Psychoanalytic Theory for Social Work Practice*. We cover some of the same issues but with different theories and case material. Reading the two books in conjunction will be a powerful learning experience.

On 14 February 2016 social work had the dubious distinction of coming top of *The Observer*'s list of stressful professions. The reasons for this must be complex, but we believe that what is missing in social work training is a theory of human nature which fits with the realities of practice. There have been various attempts to raise the status of social work, and attract students with high abilities. For example, there is now a fast-track route for students from Russell Group universities. In our view this misses the point. What social work students need is a theory of human nature which fits with the reality of what they will encounter in their practice. Able students will be the quickest to detect that they are being asked to do a job without the right tools (Anna Harvey's chapter will take this issue further).

An example

A social worker has been asked to do a home visit to a young woman with small children. The health visitor suspected her of leaving them alone at night when she goes out to get drugs. The flat is filthy and chaotic, the client is tearful. Having arrived in a hopeful mood the social worker finds her head in a whirl and feels guilty and inadequate. Experiences like this are bread and butter social work. They are part of the reason the stress levels are so high. What could make it better? First the social worker needs to recognise that her feelings of confusion and guilt are her *countertransference*. The client is projecting into her feelings she cannot tolerate. Awareness of this can restore the social worker's sense of professional competence. The social worker finds that when she talks to the mother, she cannot think about the children. This is probably because the mother cannot think about the children's needs when she feels the need for drugs.

The role of theory can be represented in a simple diagram, shown in Figure 1.1.

The client projects difficult feelings into the social worker. The social worker turns to some useful theory which gives her space to think. She can then respond to the client in a different way. This process of using theory is not easy while you are in the middle of the hurly burly of a home visit. You can turn to the triangle when you are driving back to the office or doing the washing up at home.

The next section looks in more detail at how theory can inform practice. I will then give a brief account of some of Freud's theories and some Kleinian and post-Kleinian theory. These ideas will reappear in all the other chapters of the book. There is also a list of useful texts at the end, for those who want to get to know the theory better.

Nothing so helpful as a good theory – Marion Bower

In 2015 the Conservative government pulled the financial plug on the College of Social Work. There was a great outcry from the College, but from the profession itself a resounding silence. The College had been intended to raise the status of social work. However it had half the planned membership, and I suspect many social workers felt it had no relevance for them. Social work cannot be turned into a high status profession without a body of knowledge which fits with the reality of their practice. Lawyers need a knowledge of law, doctors need a knowledge of the

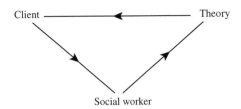

FIGURE 1.1 The role of theory in aiding social work

human body and its functions. Social workers need a knowledge of emotional development and human relationships.

I first became aware of the importance of a theoretical framework when I spent ten years organising infant/young child seminars for a post qualifying social work training. Students were expected to observe a baby or a young child once a week for ten weeks. They were asked to find a child about whom there were no concerns. In practice this meant observing babies with their mother or carer, and children in day nurseries. Students spent an hour each week observing, without making notes until afterwards. Each week the observers discussed their observations in small groups led by experienced social workers or child psychotherapists. The first thing that emerged was that most social workers were brilliant observers, and very aware of their emotional responses to the observations. The problem was that they did not have a well-developed model of human nature which would allow them to evaluate their findings. Some social workers knew about attachment theory. However in many of the nurseries children did not have an opportunity to form attachments. Their contacts with adults were fleeting even if they were ill or unhappy (obviously some nurseries were better than others). The social workers quietly sitting there 'doing nothing' were a magnet for children wanting to talk to them, show them a toy or just have a cuddle. Many of the students rated these observations and their seminars as the most helpful part of the course. Their value for many social work tasks was obvious. However when it came to writing an essay about their observations the students found it difficult. They had never been taught a theory of emotional development which fitted with their observational experience. They did not know how to interpret small children's play or use their emotional responses as a tool to evaluate the observation.

Many child protection enquiries stress that the child concerned is not *seen*. In my experience children are often *seen* but the workers do not know how to evaluate what they see. As Janet Mattinson says, 'there is nothing so helpful as a good theory'.

In one nursery, where staff were particularly unavailable, a little boy left on his own kept smiling and catching the eye of members of staff who usually smiled back. While he did this, he was building a house out of scraps of plasticine. I thought 'He is making a meal out of scraps'. From a theoretical point of view, he is in a lonely situation, but he has the capacity to build up a 'house' of adult smiles. It is likely that a child like this has helpful people in his internal world and he re-created this externally.

My next example of the value of theory is an experience I had as a social work student. My placement was in a busy teaching hospital in the Child Development unit. It dealt chiefly with diagnoses of disability in children, but some adults with a disability were also seen. My first case was a man in his early forties who had multiple sclerosis. He was currently unable to walk, but had been refusing to have a wheelchair.

Mr A and his wife were Italian. Before the onset of Mr A's disability he had been a head waiter in an Italian restaurant. Mr and Mrs A had a 16-year-old son,

Giovanni. On my first visit I rang the door. Mrs A let me in. She called Mr A from the kitchen and I was appalled when he *crawled* in. Mrs A and Giovanni complained about his stubbornness. Over a number of visits the pattern repeated itself. I made futile attempts to persuade Mr A to accept the wheelchair. On one visit I arrived and found a nun (Mr and Mrs A were Catholic). I noticed that she had been offered tea and cake, I was only given tea. 'She's a good sort of nun,' said Mrs A after she left. 'She knows the price of cabbage.' Although I was not familiar with transference I knew Mrs A felt that I did not know the price of cabbage.

My supervisor at the hospital was most amused by my lack of success. 'When you leave they will think they've driven you away.' 'Oh no,' I said, 'I've told them I'm a student on a placement.' After some thought I decided to raise this idea with Mr and Mrs A. To my surprise Mr and Mrs A beamed at me – 'of course you're leaving because we are too difficult for you. We hope you have better clients on your next job.' I was amazed at the triumph of Mr and Mrs A's feelings over the facts. Mr and Mrs A's beliefs that they were driving me away was more 'real' to them than my announcement that I was a student on a short placement. This was my first encounter with the unconscious which, up until then, had just been a theory in a book. I was also surprised to see how it cheered up Mr and Mrs A when they felt I understood them.

My supervisor's emphasis on the *transference* between me and my client is now a little old-fashioned. In fact it took place 35 years ago. Psychoanalytic theory and practice have developed since then. Now I would put more emphasis on the *countertransference* – how Mr and Mrs A made me feel. What I felt was *helpless*. I think Mr A, who had been a very active man, could not tolerate this feeling. He *projected* this feeling into his wife, and the two of them *projected* it into me. (I was a good target as I was so inexperienced.) I think if I could have reflected on this feeling I might have understood Mr A's behaviour and perhaps been able to talk to him about what lay behind it.

I was lucky to be on a course which taught psychoanalytic theory. There was a period when this was replaced by a more sociological and political view. Of course these subjects are essential, but psychoanalysis reaches the important parts of clients' minds that other theories do not reach. Psychoanalysis begins with Freud. Some of his ideas have been developed, others have been changed, but many of his concepts have had lasting value. One of these is the importance of listening very carefully to the patient/client. In social work we have learned to take what children say to us very seriously. Another of Freud's discoveries was how much of our lives are dominated by emotions which may not be conscious (like Mr and Mrs A's belief that I was leaving because they were too difficult for me). Finally Freud discovered that early experiences have a lasting impact on our personalities. This is an idea that is so widely accepted that we take it for granted.

In the next section I am going to describe the work of Freud and some of the psychoanalysts who came after him. Psychoanalysts refer to the people they treat as patients. Social workers used to refer to the people they worked with as 'clients'. Now the term 'service user' is in fashion. I think this term is an evasion. It implies the interaction between worker and client is emotionally neutral. This is blatantly not the case. Some clients can stir up very unpleasant feelings in us, such as fear or hatred. This can feel 'unprofessional'. It is not unprofessional to have these feelings – but they need to be *used professionally*. This theory will help you do this.

Freud

Freud spent all of his working life in Vienna. He started his professional life as a neurologist and made a number of interesting discoveries including the medical use of cocaine. As a Jew he found it hard to get advancement in the university so he turned to seeing patients in his private practice. Many of his early patients were Hysterics, patients who had a number of physical symptoms including paralysis which had no medical basis. The patients were often untroubled by the symptoms ('belle indifference'), although their families were upset. Up until Freud the only effective treatment was hypnosis. Freud did not like using hypnosis so he and a colleague, Josef Breuer, simply encouraged the patients to say whatever they were thinking of – *free associations*. This has relevance for social work. Very often workers see a client or family with a fixed agenda. Sometimes we can learn a lot by letting people just talk. Freud and Breuer's patients' free associations often revealed that behind the symptoms were 'forbidden' thoughts or wishes, often of a sexual nature. Freud thought that one shortcut to these forbidden thoughts was by analysing the patient's dreams. Once the patients had recounted their thoughts the symptoms usually improved. This treatment was more humane than other treatments available at the time. However it had one side effect. The patient developed an intense relationship to the doctor. One of Breuer's patients claimed she was expecting Breuer's baby (she was not, but Breuer took flight). Freud was not alarmed. He realised that the relationship with the patient could be a tool. The patient transferred on to the doctor significant figures from their childhood, for example a strict father or a depressed mother. You do not have to be a psychoanalyst to observe transference in action. The modern view is that transference permeates all relationships. Transference can colour a client's perceptions of a worker. It is not unusual for a kind and helpful social worker to be perceived as cruel by a client.

As Freud saw more and more patients he was horrified when many of them described sexual seduction by a parent or other adults. At first he was alarmed that he had discovered sexual abuse on a massive scale. After a while he decided that patients were describing wish-fulfilling fantasies. This led him to suggest that young children were sexual creatures, but their sexuality is different to adults and located in different parts of their bodies. We now know that Freud had thrown the baby out with the bathwater. Young children are being sexually abused. However Freud's concept of childhood sexuality has given us a better understanding of the impact of abuse on children's minds. It is common when talking to abused children to feel confused whether or not it really happened. This reflects the child's confusion, caused by fantasy becoming reality. Freud's work also threw light on why many children and adults who have been abused put themselves in the way of being abused again.

Freud followed the events of the First World War anxiously. He had two sons in the army. In England there was a small but growing group of psychoanalysts, some of whom were army psychiatrists. Shell shock, accompanied by a host of physical symptoms, was extremely common. Psychoanalysis gained credibility because it was the only effective and humane method of treating it. Freud was puzzled that traumatised soldiers re-lived the horrific scenes in their dreams. He called the phenomenon of revisiting a trauma *repetition compulsion*. Sometimes this meant revisiting the trauma in waking life. This can take a number of forms. It is very common for patients who have been sexually abused to put their children at risk. A research project on sexually abused girls found that some seemed to invite further abuse by behaving in a seductive manner, for example sitting with their legs apart, exposing their knickers. It is not uncommon for children who are abused to be placed with foster families, only to be abused again. This is not to blame the children. Education of foster parents about this phenomenon may help protect abused children.

Sexually abused children often feel guilt. This is not rational and they are usually told they do not need to feel this. This is not enough. Abused children often feel guilty because their childhood sexual feelings are activated, making them feel responsible. When the abuse is incestuous and the parent is of the opposite sex the child can feel guilty because Oedipal wishes have been gratified, and there is a triumph over the parent of the same sex. Freud gave the name Oedipus complex to a phase of childhood sexuality when there is a wish to 'marry' the parent of the opposite sex. In the Greek myth an oracle tells Oedipus' parents Jocasta and Laius that their son will kill his father and marry his mother. Horrified, they arrange for him to be taken away by a shepherd and left to die. The shepherd takes Oedipus away, but gives him to another king and queen. When Oedipus hears the myth as a young man he runs away from his foster parents. He meets his father at a cross-roads. They have an argument and Oedipus kills him (not realising he is his father). He carries on to a city where the sphinx is holding the inhabitants in thrall. She promises to leave if someone can answer her riddle. Oedipus answers the riddle and as a reward he gets to marry the queen (not realising it is his mother). Many years go by and Jocasta and Oedipus have children. Oedipus discovers who he is. He is horrified and puts out his eyes in remorse. Jocasta hangs herself.

There is a lot of resistance to the idea of the Oedipus complex. But it is a story which has survived for 2000 years. Do people from other cultures experience Oedipal feelings?

The Ps were an Afghan family. Father had been imprisoned for his political beliefs. He escaped and fled with his wife and their daughter to Pakistan. In Pakistan they had a baby boy. After many difficulties they came to live in England, where they had a three-bedroom flat. School were concerned that the little boy constantly drew horrific scenes and people dripping with blood. It turned out they were things his father had seen in Afghanistan before he was born. When they came to a Child and Adolescent Mental Health Services (CAMHS) service it emerged that mother had banished father to a tiny cold bedroom and taken the boy into bed with her. Mother constantly complained about a madman in the next door flat who threw his furniture out. *Unconsciously* she felt she was mad to throw out her husband. The little boy in fantasy had entered his father's traumatic experiences as well as taking his place in the parental bed.

Another way of thinking about family constellations has been described by Roger Money-Kyrle. He called it 'The Facts of Life'. These facts have a biological underpinning. Where these facts are denied, consciously or unconsciously, something is going wrong. For example paedophiles deny the significance of generational differences. These facts are: 1) the infant is totally dependant on the mother or carer, 2) generational differences exist, 3) we are all going to die.

Melanie Klein

Klein was the most revolutionary psychoanalyst since Freud. Freud expanded our awareness of childhood and the influence of early experiences on development, but he never worked directly with children. Young children cannot lie on a couch and free associate. Klein was the mother of three children. Asked to see a young child she had the idea of giving the child some of her children's toys. Klein saw play as the young child's equivalent of free associations in the adult. Over time she standardised what she offered: little people, wild and tame animals, bricks, paper, pencils, plasticine, little cars, etc. These little toys can be put in a box or basket and carried with the social worker on a home visit. By giving a child materials which do not have a ready-made story we can find out what is on a child's mind. A child will often tell the worker the story of what they are doing.

Using these materials Klein was able to work with children as young as two and a half. She opened up a world which was very different to the older child or adult. She developed the concept of an internal world. This is a world of figures based on the people we first loved and hated in life. These figures also represent aspects of ourselves. Freud had also recognised an internal world in which there was a super-ego, or conscience, based on the parents and appearing at the resolution of the Oedipus complex. We can all recognise this figure which tells us what we ought to be doing: 'You need to get that report finished!' Klein discovered that there was a much earlier version of the superego which was harsh and cruel – an expression of the child's sadism. Klein found that young children have very intense loving and hating feelings. From very early on the child wants to take in good experiences and get rid of bad ones. This process is based on the child's physical experiences of feeding and excreting. Getting rid of bad experiences is not something a child can do in reality, but it can do it in phantasy. Klein called this process *projective identification*. In phantasy the child *projects* the bad self or experience and the mother becomes *identified* with the bad self. This concept can explain many difficult experiences in social work.

A client feels hatred of a social worker who has come to investigate a child protection concern. Through projective identification the social worker becomes *the* hating person. An unpleasant experience for a kind and helpful social worker.

Freud's schema of development was a sexual one: Oral, Anal, Phallic and Genital. He thought that there could be problems if we regress to an earlier stage. Klein's schema was different. She thought in terms of positions which we oscillate between throughout life.

The *paranoid schizoid position* occupies roughly the first three months of life; however the baby continues to use projective identification, not only to get rid of bad experiences, but also to communicate. This is something we all do throughout life. Although Klein stressed this was a phantasy, Klein's patient Wilfred Bion pointed out that it can have a real effect on the recipient. Anyone who has listened to a baby cry in a supermarket will know what he means. The paranoid schizoid position gets rather a bad press, but it is very important as it is the point we begin to sort out good from bad experiences. If a child is overwhelmed by bad experiences this sorting out is difficult and a state of confusion can develop.

As the child develops it becomes aware that the 'bad' mother it hates is the same as the 'good' mother it loves. This leads to feelings of guilt and sadness and a wish to make reparation. If these feelings are too painful to be borne the child resorts to defences, particularly the *manic defence*. In this state of mind there is a feeling of being powerful and that individuals do not matter. This feeling is expressed in many computer games, where there are all-powerful figures and the world is sharply divided into good and bad. There is no space for vulnerability, dependency or complexity. Freud's line of development is a one-way street, although there can be regressions to earlier states. These are pathological. The Kleinian line of development oscillates between paranoid schizoid and depressive as part of normal development. Projective identification and manic defences are used by all of us some of the time. These positions and defences are also a useful way of thinking about social work practices and institutions. Most social workers come into social work to put things right for people. They want to make reparation to their internal and external objects. Practical experience reveals that many of the people social workers deal with are very damaged by what has happened to them and not easily 'put right'. Often there is a regression to the paranoid schizoid position with its worries about 'covering yourself' or 'minding your back'. Child Protection Plans are notoriously unrealistic and omnipotent in tone. They are expressions of a manic defence which denies the extent of the emotional damage.

This may seem a rather gloomy state of affairs. However, surely it is better to set realistic goals for our work and have the satisfaction of achieving them. When I was working for Social Services there were some families who had a social worker for most of their childbearing years. It was an acknowledgement that there would be little change, but a belief that social work support would make enough of a difference. Nowadays there is little opportunity for this sort of work but there are still important services that social workers can provide. What all our clients need is *understanding*. By this I mean the special sort of understanding described by Wilfred Bion, which he called *containment*.

Bion was a tank commander in the First World War. This was a horrific job. If a tank was hit by shells it could go up in flames, frying everyone inside. Bion said that 'a tank commander does not need to be clever but they need to be able to think under fire'. This is what social workers need to do from the emotional point of view. Bion called this capacity *containment*. It originates in the mother's relationship with the baby. The baby projects unbearable feelings into the mother. The mother is disturbed by these feelings, but unlike the baby she has (hopefully) the capacity to process the feelings and return them to the baby in a more digested form. Over time the baby internalises the mother's capacity for containment.

This is the ideal state of affairs. However many of our clients have not been emotionally contained by their mother; in fact they may have been used as receptacles for parental projections of violence, sexuality or depression. If they meet a containing person they take full advantage of this. It is common to do a home visit feeling quite all right and come out feeling disheartened, confused or guilty. Your clients probably feel better. Clients can be aware that you are tolerating projections from them. When I ran a group for depressed mothers one of them said 'All your plants are dying, it must be our noxious fumes'.

Ideally social workers should have supervision about their work with clients. Unfortunately much supervision is managerial, which is important, but does not develop your capacity for face-to-face work. An important tool for self-supervision is the *process recording*. In this you will write down everything that happens in the interview. What is said, who does what and how you feel. A common feeling in child protection cases is guilt, not by the client, but by the social worker. The client probably feels a sense of persecution by the child and the worker. Guilt is projected into the social worker who has the capacity to feel it. This is not to say that workers and departments never make mistakes or let a client down. But this guilt is usually acknowledged. There are times when clients feel that the worker is letting them down. This is when the worker goes on holiday or leaves the department. As many of our clients have had traumatic losses or separations, it is not surprising that they feel hurt when a social worker leaves them, or afraid they have been too much for the worker. (See my example of Mr A on p. 3.) It is common practice to bring along the new worker to introduce them. In my view this does not help anyone. What the client needs is an opportunity to express what they feel about the worker leaving. As my experience with Mr and Mrs A shows, it is a relief for clients to be able to say what they think. I took over the M family from a much older colleague. I left the department six months later and felt very guilty about this. Mr M said 'You're the best social worker we've had!' I asked why and he said 'You don't call me Billy!' This may seem trivial, but if someone feels inadequate (as this man did) they appreciate being treated as an adult. It shows respect. 'John hit Mary and Jane screamed at them to stop it.' Hearing this report at a case conference I found it impossible to tell who were the parents and who were the children. Many people we see have difficulties in establishing generation barriers. The language we use can help.

Social workers doing infant/child observations often find that the child is also observing *them*. Clients are quick to pick up that a worker wants to be seen to be friendly or can be easily seduced. This can be a small thing, but it can also be a key moment in a child protection tragedy.

Registering change/making change

As we all know from personal experience making changes in ourselves is very difficult. However as social workers we are there to try and change people's lives for the better, but if we are unrealistic in what we expect we can get disheartened. The psychoanalyst Ron Britton has suggested that we aim for small but necessary steps. This could simply be a parent feeling able to sit through a court hearing. Andrew Cooper's chapter describes a lonely man who finally manages to acknowledge to his social worker that he feels suicidal. This is a significant step, as the social worker can plan regular visits to help him talk about this, and also possibly arrange an assessment by a psychiatrist. Many people use their children as receptacles for unwanted feelings of their own. If the parent gets help from a social worker to re-own these feelings their relationship with their child can improve. For example, one mother described her son as 'the aggressive one'. In reality she was very hostile to the social worker. The social worker was able to tolerate this. The mother then referred to the boy as 'my most affectionate child'.

Change does not go in a straight line. Getting better can make things feel worse. Parents who reduce their drug intake can become aware of the damage it has done to their children. This may send them back to drugs to blot out this knowledge. One aspect of change is that it takes time, but spending time with a client can bring about change. Ideally it is best to see a client or family on a regular day or at a regular time. If you are forced to change the time it is a good idea to offer another. Many social work clients have been starved of attention when they were young. Just the presence of a receptive person is therapeutic.

2

CONTEXT

Navigating contested professional identities in difficult times

James Blewett

This book attempts to apply psychodynamic theory to real world social work practice. Its premise is that these ideas can make sense of, and provide strategies for managing, the highly complex social problems in a relational context that families and therefore social work practitioners face. Social work however is not a profession that can easily be fitted within a single definition. It is a professional identity that is characterised by its highly fluid and multifaceted nature. Social workers have a number of different, apparently contradictory roles that as practitioners they are often asked to implement simultaneously. The nature of these roles and the balance between these respective tasks have been, and continue to be, highly contested. Moreover, the profession has an often-uneasy relationship with the drivers of social policy and therefore can, in certain respects, become highly politicised. In this period in which the UK faces, in a climate of considerable uncertainty, so many economic and social challenges, settling on a clear perspective on the role of social work is particularly difficult.

This chapter will attempt to engage with this debate. It will provide a brief overview of the development of the profession and the debates regarding the definition of social work. In so doing it will explore the different roles of social work and the discussions around the profession's identity. The chapter will then focus on some of the current challenges facing practitioners and consider the prospects for the profession in these difficult times. The chapter will also seek to locate use of psychodynamic theory in a wider and historical context.

Defining social work: why the perennial debate?

Historically social work has been the subject to a regular debate about its roles and tasks (Seebohm, 1968; Barclay, 1982; Department of Health and Department for

Education and Skills, 2006; General Social Care Council, 2008; Department for Education, 2014a, 2014b). Other professions are also subject to debate and reflection but social work seems to be subject of a uniquely continuous and at times existential debate about its identity. Why is this the case? Perhaps it is because a social worker is in a much more fluid role than, for example, a teacher or doctor. Complicated and challenging as those jobs undoubtedly are, they are working within a relatively clearly defined professional space. While there might be very robust debates about *how* they occupy that professional space the fact that teachers, for example, are focused on educating children is uncontested. Social workers on the other hand undertake a multitude of roles. These range from the practical, to the socio-legal and the therapeutic. The basis of the debates regarding social work extend beyond the complexity of the social work task. It is also because of the relationship that social work has to social policy. Social work in the UK is largely about the way in which the state intervenes in the private lives of its citizens. In the field of children and families this has been about how people raise their children, the respective rights of children and their parents, and support that they may expect from the state. The nature of rights and expectations of the role of the state have been at the heart of the debate regarding social work's identity. Exploring child welfare more broadly Fox Harding (1997), in her seminal analysis, identified four historic traditions which relate to these questions:

a. *Laissez-faire and patriarchy.* This is the position that supports only minimal state intervention in the private life of the family. The state's role should be minimal and seen as almost inherently intrusive. Intervention should only take place where there are very clear concerns regarding child safety. Fox Harding linked this to patriarchy as this libertarian position on the state was often accompanied by a normative and somewhat idealised view of traditional family life in the nuclear family.

b. *State paternalism and child protection.* This tradition in child welfare supports extensive state intervention in some (often poorer) families' lives. The state is perceived as essentially benign and its role is to 'rescue' children from poor parenting. The negative effects of state intervention such as the danger of punitive and unnecessary intrusions into families' lives tend to be minimised and structural factors that contribute to inadequate care overlooked.

c. *The modern defence of the birth family and parents' rights.* This position also supports extensive state intervention but believes that state intervention should be primarily supportive, with the provision of early help and family support. Coercive intervention should be at much higher thresholds than those who supported the previous position and if children are taken into state care then links with birth families should be preserved.

d. *Children's rights and child liberation.* This position considers children to be autonomous citizens with full civil rights, with an equivalence with adults. The concept of parental rights and state activity in this area is treated with scepticism and the primary focus is on the child's perspective, their wishes and feelings.

Each of these positions will have implications for the role of social work in terms of its activity but more generally where social workers are located within the welfare system.

Social work: three broad traditions

Social work has been carried out in many different places and with many different groups. However, Payne (2014: 13) identifies three historic models for the role of social work. These are: Therapeutic; Maintenance; and Transformational.

The **therapeutic tradition** is that which is most closely associated with psychodynamic ideas (Bower, 2005). It is based on the belief that social workers need to understand the impact of the inner world on family members they are working with. Social workers need a sophisticated understanding of the impact of families' psycho-social histories. As Howe argues,

> the complex interplay between the past and the present, the psychological inside and the social outside, is the dance that practitioners have to understand if they are to make sense of what is going on and intervene appropriately and effectively in people's lives.
>
> *(Howe et al., 1999)*

This tradition is most closely associated with relationship based practice (Ruch, 2013) in which there has been renewed interest amongst both social workers and policy makers and will be discussed further below.

The **maintenance** tradition is that which is most closely associated with statutory social work. Within this model social workers are both experts and the gatekeepers of resources (Murphy, 2004). Working within a complex legal structure, social workers undertake a number of key tasks on behalf of society with regard to child welfare. For example, social workers will assess whether children are being maltreated and the possible harm to children (Calder, 2013). They will also assess need and access appropriate resources on the family's behalf as well as providing information and advice. In respect of the children looked after by the state, social workers will be key in coordinating the 'corporate parenting' role of the local authority.

The **emancipatory** position reflects social work's radical tradition. It is based upon a structural analysis of society in which families' experiences and outcomes are powerfully influenced by factors such as poverty, racism and gender inequality (Dominelli, 2002). As well as having implications for how social workers understand a family's needs, it also has implications for how workers approach and build relationships with families. It also raises important questions about where social workers are located, how services are designed, as well as how they practise. For example, this tradition informs some of the new ways of working that social workers are adopting and that will be discussed later in this chapter (Featherstone et al., 2014).

There are limitations to any attempt to categorise the rich traditions of social work and its associated disciplines into three distinct categories. A current influential theorist such as Ferguson (2016), for example, writes extensively about statutory social work, drawing on both psychodynamic ideas as well as critical sociological theory. More generally many of those influenced by psychodynamic ideas would argue that it is a caricature of their position to describe them as not interested in the impact of either the environment or wider structural factors. Similarly, those arguing from an emancipatory perspective would argue that it is a gross simplification of their position to suggest that they are not interested in the psychological and emotional world of an individual or family seeking help.

It is therefore more accurate to understand these three models as three dimensions within a single model of social work (represented in Figure 2.1 as three points on a triangle). Payne (2014) stresses the on-going dynamic tension between these three dimensions, and that they are not mutually exclusive. The prevailing model within any social work context will be largely determined by the political and organisational imperatives of the agency in which social workers are employed. That is not to say that individual practitioners do not aspire to work in a reflective, relationship based way (Banks 2006; Munro 2004) However inevitably a social worker attached to a service-user led voluntary sector project will have much greater opportunity to apply professional discretion, at least in the short term, than a children and family social worker in a local authority assessment team.

These ideas had been anticipated by Halmos (1965), who, for example, noted when reviewing workforce data from the 1950s that social workers tended to be defined by *who they worked for* rather than always *what they actually did*. If this was the case 50 years ago then this has been even more the case in the more recent past. For many years *being a social worker* has tended to be synonymous with *working for a local authority social services department*.

Many typologies of the role of social work have been proposed over the last 50 years (see for example, Sheldon 1978; Hanvey & Philpot 1994; Gambrill 1994; Payne 2006), all of which are to some degree complementary.

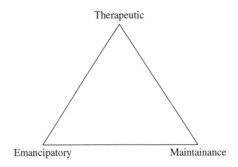

FIGURE 2.1 Three models of social work

Successive definitions revisit common components. A review of *The tasks and roles of social workers* carried out for the Scottish Executive (Asquith et al., 2005) concluded that social work has been seen to incorporate all the following tasks:

- counsellor or caseworker;
- advocate;
- assessor of risk and of need;
- care manager;
- agent of social control.

(paras 5.5–5.15)

The key point that Asquith et al. were making is that social workers are often undertaking all five of these roles with families simultaneously. This is what makes the job of social worker complex, challenging and at times infuriating, but also ultimately very rewarding. The social worker needs to understand risk and safety in families, advocate on their behalf, but then on occasions work against their wishes.

However, as we indicated at the outset, any adequate understanding of the roles and tasks of social work must take account of the interlocking nature of values, principles *and* tasks. A number of core *principles* have been identified as underpinning social work, but are in reality they also serve as definitions:

- It is a problem-solving activity.
- The focus is on the whole of a person's/family's life, their social support network, their neighbourhood and community.
- The value system is based on human and civil rights.
- The social model is the framework for practice.
- Social workers work with individuals, families, groups or communities to define together the outcomes they are seeking.
- The process and the relationship are a core part of the service and can represent a service in itself.
- The purpose of social work is to increase the life chances and opportunities of people using services by building on their strengths, expertise and experience to maximise their capacities.

(Brand et al., 2005: 2–3)

Asquith et al. (2005) argued there was no unanimity as to *what social work* is. They concluded that:

- There are competing definitions of social work.
- Social work has several wider social functions.
- The function of social work is highly contested.
- Social work plays an important function in social integration.
- Social work may fulfil a social control function.
- Social work is expected to address the failure of social policies.

(para 3.17)

The author and colleagues were asked by the General Social Care Council (GSCC) and the Social Care Institute for Excellence (SCIE) to explore seven core components:

1.   Understanding the dynamic between the individual and the social
2.   Social work and social justice
3.   The transformatory significance of the relationship
4.   The enabling role of social work
5.   The therapeutic role of social work
6.   The management of risk to both the community and the individual
7.   The evidence base for social work practice

(Blewett et al., 2008)

Social work and the era of reform

An emerging consensus

In October 2008, *The Sun* newspaper highlighted the death of a toddler, Peter Connolly, in north London. Its coverage included a scathing attack on the professionals involved who it believed had 'failed Baby P' (Jones, 2014). It created, as so many children's deaths have in the past, a heightened political debate in which the director of children's services of the local authority lost her job, and there was another period of intense national debate about the efficacy of social work. Interestingly other professionals were criticised such as the paediatrician and GP, but these criticisms did not provoke the same national debate about their professions.

Besides the immediate furore the Labour government also instituted an urgent review into the state of the social work profession, the Social Work Taskforce. This drew together a broad range of social work professionals, senior managers and academics and was chaired by an ex-director of children's services, Moira Gibb. Her review carried out in 2009 and early 2010 concluded that many social workers had caseloads that were too high, that the quality of supervision was often not good enough, that administrative systems were cumbersome and IT inefficient (Department for Education, 2009). The Taskforce produced a range of recommendations that concluded in the creation of chief social work posts, principal social workers in each locality, an assessed and supported year for newly qualified social workers, national standards for supervision and workload, and the creation of a College of Social Work. It also proposed a new conceptual framework for understanding both social workers' professional identity but also within a career-long framework. This was entitled the Professional Capabilities Framework (PCF) and attempted to move social work away from the competency based assessment upon which it had been based for the last twenty years. It was argued that such a competency based approach had produced a somewhat mechanical 'tick box' approach to social work professional development and assessment.

These capabilities seek to synthesise knowledge, values and skills and recognise that the knowledge and skills needed for social work are changing. PCF was to be managed and maintained by the newly created College of Social Work.

There was widespread and positive consensus around these proposed reforms and the Social Work Taskforce evolved into the Social Work Reform Board tasked with implementing the reform programme. In May 2010, however, there was a change of government with the Coalition (of Conservatives and Liberal Democrats) replacing the Labour government. The new government supported the ongoing work of the Reform Board but political attention was now focused on a new initiative. The children minister at the time, Tim Loughton, asked Professor Eileen Munro of the LSE to undertake a review of the child protection system.

Munro carried out her review from 2010–2012 and produced four reports (Munro, 2010, 2011a, 2011b, 2012). Many of her conclusions were similar to those of the Social Work Task Force and her recommendations were both congruent and complementary. Munro based her analysis on the work of systems theorists such as Wood and Reason who had tried to understand how error and failures could occur in systems as diverse as health and the air accident industry. Munro (2011a, 2011b) argued that child protection was inherently uncertain and anxiety providing, requiring professionals (particularly social workers) to manage rather than eradicate risk. She argued that the traditional response to this had been the techno-managerialist methods. This sought to place practitioners under great scrutiny, to remove the human factor wherever possible and to place individual workers and managers under greater pressure to perform better. The result was that the administrative system for child care practice had become highly bureaucratic and complicated, with high levels of managerial scrutiny throughout. This had, Munro argued, produced a professional culture that 'hobbled' rather than promoted the expertise of practitioners. *In seeking to create greater safety the way that the system had developed had inadvertently undermined professional judgement, discretion and the capacity to think clearly.*

An analogy (not used by Munro herself) might be a car SATNAV system. The equipment is of course designed to help drivers navigate the road system. Certainly, it can provide assistance but there is a danger that drivers become solely reliant upon the tool and do not develop their own 'practice wisdom' of using their judgement regarding the best routes. Moreover, these small boxes attached to the dashboard can provide so much information that it is tempting to become distracted and focus on the SATNAV rather than the road. Similarly, Munro argued that social workers could become focused on procedural compliance, of 'doing things right' rather than focusing on the child or young person and their family 'the right thing'.

Munro therefore came to similar conclusions as the Social Work Taskforce. She argued that social workers needed manageable workloads and access to high quality supervision and endorsed many of the proposals of the Taskforce such as the creation of principle social work posts and the development of a robust Assessed and Supported Year in Employment (ASYE) national programme. Munro also recommended that greater emphasis be placed on services that could offer early help and that greater attention be paid to the perennial challenge of poor communication between agencies. Munro argued that national inspection, regulatory and performance frameworks should not focus so much on timescales but on some of the harder-to-measure areas such as the 'child's journey' through the child welfare system.

The 'reforms' of 2010–2012 however were taking places against a difficult budgetary backdrop and were only part of a series of reviews and changes taking places at national governmental level. Field (2011) was asked to undertake a review of poverty; Tickell (2011) of early years; and Norgrove (2011) of the family justice system. This latter review had an impact on social work practice, recommending that care proceedings should be speeded up and take place within a twenty-six-week time limit. The constraint on budgets meant that there were significant cuts in both local authorities' services and those of their partner agencies. The language and strategy of austerity went much further than simply cutting services. Benefit 'reform' involved very significant cuts in the income of large numbers of poorer families, and also an increasingly punitive view by ministers of those on benefits being responsible for their own plight, that there was a culture in the country of benefit dependency, and a growing divide between those perceived to be 'deserving' as opposed to 'undeserving' poor. George Osborne, the chancellor in this period, went as far as to suggest that the death of five children following their father setting fire to their house was the result of a 'benefits culture'. The Trussell Trust (2012) reported a huge growth in the demand for foodbanks.

The Troubled Families Initiative also reinforced this perspective. Introduced in the aftermath of a series of riots that occurred in the summer of 2011, this attempted to 'turn around' the 'most troubled families' through a combination of family support but also 'tough love'. The implication of this project was that social workers were too soft. A new better type of project worker would be recruited who would succeed where social workers failed. In reality a recent evaluation of this project showed it had failed in its aims.

Another result of austerity had been what the new Coalition government had described as a 'bonfire of the quangos' as they sought to rein in spending on what was described as a bloated public sector. Two casualties of this process were the GSCC, the still relatively new social work regulator, and the Children's Workforce Development Council, which had overseen many of the early reforms in childcare social work.

A narrative of failure

Parton (2016) argues that this period of consensus regarding social work reform began to change in approximately 2013. At this time, there were a series of serious case reviews (Pelka; Khan; Rotherham) that ministers argued provided further evidence of the failure of the child protection system in general and social work professionals in particular. There were also a number of damning reports by the inspection agency Ofsted, most notably in Doncaster, Birmingham and Slough. With their conclusions captured in single broad labels of 'inadequate', 'requires improvement', 'good' or 'outstanding' they could consign local authorities (in the case of the two negative categories) to periods of uncertainty, instability and a downward spiral of staff morale. The response to the negative inspections in each of the named local authorities was to take children's services away from direct local authority control and establish an independent children's trust.

It was around this time, in 2013, that Sir Martin Narey was asked to undertake a review of social work education, and he reported in early 2014. The basis of this review was a belief amongst ministers that social work education was not sufficiently preparing social workers for practice. Interestingly, a completely separate review of social work education for the adults' services sector was undertaken by Professor Croisdale Appleby. Narey concluded (2014) that social work education did indeed have some flaws. In a report that was based on a series of interviews and included some observations made on and from social media he expressed a view that, rather than preparing social work students for the reality of statutory child care social work, current social work training was dominated by radical academics who focused on teaching anti-oppressive practice (the aforementioned caricature of the emancipatory position). He made no significant reference to the PCF and instead argued that there was an absence of a clear statement as to what social workers should know and what skills they should possess to carry out their role. Narey argued that the profession needed such a statement. He also criticised what he concluded was weak regulation of social work education and argued that the Health and Care Professionals Council, which had taken over the regulation of social workers after the demise of the GSCC, did not have the specialist skills and capacity to carry out this function, and that there should be a specific new regulator for social work. Narey also endorsed emerging 'fast track' training programmes, which he believed would attract new talent and a new generation of 'practice leaders', given their targeting of graduates from Russell Group universities (see Chapter 5, by Anna Harvey and Fiona Henderson).

The report was welcomed by government and the new Chief Social Worker and within the next six months a new Knowledge and Skills Statement was produced for social workers undertaking statutory roles (Department for Education, 2014a). These were criticised (Department for Education, 2014a, 2014b) for having a very narrow definition of 'statutory' and also that there was no reference to the values of social work. The response of the Department for Education was that these areas were covered in what they believed to be the complementary PCF.

Nicky Morgan, the then Education Secretary, announced that the Knowledge and Skills Statements were to going to be used as the basis for assessing all social workers (and ultimately their managers) who worked in statutory roles. This assessment was going to be the basis for accreditation and a newly approved child and family practitioner role. The rationale for this accreditation process was to restore and promote the 'public's faith' in the social work profession, which the government felt was necessary. A measure of how necessary the government felt this to be was contained in a speech by then prime minister David Cameron in 2015. Having asked for a standing ovation for social workers in his party conference speech in 2013, two year later he took a much more critical line. He pointed out that the poor outcomes for young people in the care system are tragically unsatisfactory. While social workers must take some responsibility for this, Cameron seemed unaware that most children are severely emotionally troubled before they come into care, and the government is not willing to spend the sort of money that would make a difference.

Morgan also announced that 'reform' would be promoted through the establishment of an Innovation Fund. This involved substantial, although strictly time-limited, amounts of new funding for specific projects in local authorities. What has characterised many of the projects under the auspices of social work reform is that they have utilised approaches drawn from behavioural psychology (Scott et al., 2012) and systems theory (Turnell and Edwards, 1999).

The current challenges facing children's and families' social workers

Social work with children and families therefore finds itself in a somewhat paradoxical position in that there is a government narrative of aspiration and reform but against a backdrop of very real pressures and difficulties. This final section of this chapter focuses on five key challenges that the profession must currently negotiate.

A system under pressure

The policies of 'austerity' which have dominated domestic policy in the UK for nearly a decade have seen a significant reduction in the size and scope of the welfare state (Johnstone, 2016). Indeed there is no sign of this process lessening in the coming years with the sector facing a period of further uncertainty and contraction (Crewe, 2016). This not only impacts on local government where most children and families' social workers still work but also the NHS and the voluntary sector. This is not, of course, the first period of financial constraint, and indeed managing the tension between the family's needs and the resources that are available is a perennial feature of children and families' social work. Nevertheless most commentators agree the cuts in budgets in recent years are qualitatively different (Hastings et al., 2015; Crewe, 2016). Estimates put the level of cuts to local government in general and social care specifically at between 40 and 60 per cent. This has not only led to a severe contraction of the state but also to a weakening of the 'ecosystem' of family support. Many agencies that potentially make up the support packages for children in the children social care system (e.g. in public care, on child protection plans or children in need plans) have lost resources and have significantly diminished capacity. Youth services and CAMHS are striking examples of this. However, austerity also impacts on families and communities. Changes to the benefit system, for example, in conjunction with a low wage insecure economy have undermined the social capital (Webber et al., 2015) and therefore resilience of many families in the community who are in most need of support (Hastings et al., 2015).

The 'perfect storm' that social work services have had to manage is that in the context of this pressure on resources there has been a significant growth in demand since the Peter Connolly story was publicised in 2008. Surges in referrals to children's services following child deaths are not uncommon. On other occasions, after the publicity has receded, the rates of demand have returned to pre-crisis levels. In this case it has not, with a rise of 79 per cent in referrals between 2008 and 2015 and the number of children in care rising from approximately 60,000 to 69,540 in the same period.

A negative context for practice

It is perhaps all the more galling for many practitioners that in the context of having to manage this 'perfect storm' and of striving to provide high quality services they have had to face much ongoing criticism.

The social work profession should avoid being defensive about its practice and recognise that the consequences of poor practice can be dire and in some instances detrimentally life-changing. Nevertheless a 'reform' agenda which does not acknowledge the impact of austerity is not only unfair but runs the risk of overlooking some of the very real causes that underpin the challenges that have been widely acknowledged since the Social Work Task Force and the Munro Review of Child Protection

'New' ways of working and the social work profession

It is in this context that the 'new' ways of working that have been increasingly popular in social work have been introduced. As was argued above many of these new approaches are drawn from other disciplines and indeed are not particularly new. Signs of Safety is nearly twenty years old and other popular approaches such as motivational interviewing and many of the behavioural and systemic methods are well established. Certainly they have often proven popular with practitioners (Bunn, 2013) and appear to have stimulated genuine interest in improving practice and an exploration for finding new ways of working with families.

There are, however, two important potential pitfalls with such an approach. The first is the danger of seeing a 'new' way of working as a 'silver bullet'. That is, it can reinforce a belief (or perhaps hope) that there is a single solution to highly complex social situations in which social workers are required to intervene. Furthermore, the focus on skills and often manualised approaches can down play the central role that professional values and ethics play in understanding and intervening in the private lives of families. Secondly, it can undermine the profession's identity and risk overlooking the achievements of social work. It can feed the negative narrative that social work must be rescued in some way by adopting techniques and professional cultural features associated with other professional groups, most notably psychology and family therapy. On the contrary, as was argued earlier in this chapter, one of the striking features of social work is the pluralistic knowledge-base upon which it is founded.

Understanding the needs of children and their carers: a child focused system?

Given the challenging professional environment which social work now faces a strong sense of professional value base and sense of professional identity are crucial. The motivation is not (what could be perceived as) a professionally parochial idea of 'protecting social work'. A strong social work profession is uniquely placed to deliver child-centred practice that is not built upon a belief that in some sense children's welfare is more important than treating parents ethically and sensitively. While the Children Act 1989 is premised on the welfare of the child being paramount it also recognised that the most effective way of promoting the welfare and safeguarding children is to support their parents.

This recognition of the central role of family support across the continuum of need including those children in need of protection has been long recognised (Tunstill et al., 2006; Blewett, 2010; Featherstone et al., 2014). Indeed internationally Tobis (2013) argues, on the basis of the New York child welfare system, that child welfare systems work most effectively when parents are treated as 'partners rather than pariahs'. That is not to say that social workers will not be in positions where they have to have extremely difficult discussions with parents on some occasions and take actions which are directly opposed to the parents' wishes and preferences. Rather it recognises the importance of a relationship based practice that does put the child or young person at the heart of practice while also treating parental views respectfully. Moreover, such a position is also based on recognising the multiple form of discrimination that families can face in their lives. Wilkins and Boahen (2013) argue that rigorous analytical mindset is based upon self-criticism, respectful curiosity and listening to the views of service users including when they are unhappy with the position social workers are taking.

The need for 'professional resilience'

In order to realise this aspiration of social work practice that supports families, is child-focused and fundamentally humane, social workers both individually and collectively must be in a position whereby they can withstand the wider pressures and challenges that have been articulated throughout this chapter. They therefore need a level of professional resilience. Grant and Kinman (2014) argue that professional resilience in social work is threefold:

- ability to manage stress and adversity;
- ability to adjust to changing situations;
- self-awareness; the ability to reflect.

The social work reform agenda has, to a degree, reflected this. It has been widely acknowledged that the 'stress and adversity' must be realistically manageable and that social workers should have caseloads that are reasonable and proportionate to their experience. Also, it has been recognised that access to high quality supervision is crucial (Carpenter et al., 2012). Not only is it an important arena in which the quality of practice is monitored and quality assured but it is also where workers' anxiety can be contained, their self-awareness raised, and that authoritative person-centred practice can be modelled.

Such a 'tone' can only be set in supervision if it is modelled across the organisations in which social workers are located. Leadership therefore plays a key role in social work agencies. Clear managerial direction is important, but a vital component of this is ensuring that workers are connected to the people around them. This is no easy task, not only because of the challenges outlined above but also because large open-plan offices and the increasing use of remote working makes maintaining supportive professional relationships difficult at times (Broadhurst and Mason, 2014). The leadership rising to this challenge is essential if individual practitioners are to be enabled to provide the high-quality care that children and their families need.

Conclusion

This chapter has outlined many of the challenges that the social work profession currently faces. Many of these challenges are formidable, particularly in the context of austerity, as diminished resources are combined with ideological critiques of the profession and its efficacy in supporting children and their families. However, rising to and meeting such challenges is not new for the profession and in many senses social work's development has been driven by responses to attacks on its credibility. Throughout the remainder of this book there will be examples of excellent social work practice and indeed this reflects the fine work that is happening all over the country every day of the week. Perhaps the most fundamental challenge for social work is to find a national voice that can articulate these achievements and offer a constructive but robust response to the critiques of the profession. This is not only for the sake of social worker practitioners but also for the families and communities the profession seeks to serve.

Editors' afterword

This chapter provides important insight into social work practice and training today. It also describes how social work looks in several important reports on the profession. What comes across immediately is the *complexity* of the task. A social worker may be expected to support a parent *and* take their child into care. This illustrates one of the most enduring dichotomies – that of *care and control*. A closer examination of the social work task in reality shows that apparent contradictions are different aspects of the same task. It is not 'kind' to allow parents to abuse their children, and a social worker may be the best professional to enable parents to mourn the loss of a child. A social worker who worked in an assessment centre, which was the last-chance saloon, told me that even when the children were taken away, the parents were happy to keep coming three or even five times a week. Ironically this humane practice would have an element of social control, because parents who have a chance to mourn are less likely to have a replacement child, or are more able to look after their child if they do. This is an example of how an understanding of psychological processes can underpin both care and control.

There is a cliché that social workers are too much about caring and not enough about control. Following the riots of 2011 the Conservative government set up a 'Troubled Families Initiative' under the direction of Louise Casey. This recruited robust individuals who were not social workers. Needless to say, part of the motivation for this project was to get people off benefits. Louise Casey praised her staff's directness. 'They were not afraid to intervene in the private lives of their clients if they thought it was necessary. "You know your kids are going to be taken away if you don't do something about this fella [violent partner]."' The implication is 'let's not have any of this wishy-washy social work understanding'. Of course any experienced social worker knows that women who leave violent partners often hook up with another one. Ever since the first women's refuge opened in Chiswick, it has been known that when women separate from violent men, they can be violent towards their own children. Not surprisingly it has recently been announced that the Troubled Families Initiative has not met its own goals.

At the same time there is justice in the idea that social workers are not adequately prepared for their roles. When social work gave up on psychoanalytic theory there was a vacuum where a realistic theory of human development and behaviour should be. Gradually courses put more emphasis on ethics and anti-oppressive practice as if they were theories of human development. Psychoanalytic theory has been creeping back via attachment theory and relationship-based social work. These have been developed in academic environments and are often confusingly mixed together, without the darker and more disturbing aspects of psychoanalysis that are so helpful in difficult cases. For example, psychoanalysis can explain why clients may spoil a helpful intervention.

The reason that we need to face the darker side of human nature is that we must accept that some clients are so disturbed or damaged by their experiences that they cannot be 'put right'. It is difficult to describe the level of trauma and misery that lie behind these figures. Some of these young people will be too emotionally damaged to be restored to an ordinary life. This is the hidden fear that lies behind every social work intervention. Although we believe that psychoanalytically informed interventions are the most effective for young people like this, we are also aware that they need jobs, housing or benefits – that new dirty word. As a society we have turned against our most vulnerable members.

Like most people who go into the helping professions, social workers want to put right damaged people in their internal world by putting people right in the external world. We think the difficulty of doing this is one reason why social workers leave the profession. Understanding psychoanalytic theory helps us identify small but meaningful changes. It also makes the work *interesting*.

References

Asquith, S., Clark, C. and Waterhouse, L. (2005) *The Role of the Social Worker in the 21st Century*. Edinburgh: Scottish Executive.

Banks, S. (2006) *Ethics and Values in Social Work*. London: Palgrave Macmillan.

Barclay, P.M. (chair) (1982) *Social Workers: Their Role and Tasks*. London: Bedford Square Press.

Blewett, J. (2010) Reflections on the impact of Children Act 1989: child care policy, the knowledge base and the evolving role of social work. *Journal of Children's Services*.

Blewett, J., Lewis, J. and Tunstill, J. (2008) *The Changing Roles and Tasks of Social Work: A Literature Informed Discussion Paper*. London: General Social Care Council.

Bower, M. (ed.) (2005) *Psychoanalytic Theory for Social Work Practice*. London: Routledge.

Brand, D., Reith, T. and Statham, D. (2005) *Core Roles and Tasks of Social Workers. A Scoping Study for the GSCC*. London: General Social Care Council

Broadhurst, K. and Mason, C. (2014) Social work beyond the VDU: foregrounding co-presence in situated practice – why face-to-face practice matters. *British Journal of Social Work* 44(3), 578–595.

Bunn, A. (2013) *Signs of Safety® in England*. London: National Society for the Prevention of Cruelty to Children.

Calder, M.C. (2013) Risk & child protection: triangulation, trials & templates. In Calder, M.C. and Hackett, S. (eds) *Assessments in Child Care: Volume 2. Theory, Research and Practice Applications*. Dorset: Russell House Publishing.

Carpenter, J., Webb, C., Bostock, L. and Coomber, C. (2012) Effective supervision in social work and social care. *SCIE Research Briefing* 43. London: Social Care Institute of Excellence.

Crewe, T. (2016) The strange death of municipal England. *London Review of Books* 38(24), 6–10.

Department of Health and Department for Education and Skills (2006) *Options for Excellence: Building the Social Care Workforce for the Future*. London: The Stationery Office.

Department for Education (2009) *Building a Safe, Confident Future – The Final Report of the Social Work Task Force*. London: The Stationery Office.

Department for Education (2014a) *Knowledge and Skills statement for children and families social workers*. London: The Stationery Office.

Department for Education (2014b) *Putting Children First: Delivering Our Vision for Excellent Children's Social Care*. London: The Stationery Office.

Dominelli, L. (2002) *Anti Oppressive Social Work Theory and Practice*. Basingstoke, Hampshire: Palgrave Macmillan.

Featherstone, B., Morris, K. and White, S. (2014) *Re-Imagining Child Protection – Towards Humane Social Work with Families*. Bristol: Policy Press.

Ferguson, H. (2016) Researching social work practice close up: Using ethnographic and mobile methods to understand encounters between social workers, children and families. *British Journal of Social Work* 46(1), 153–168.

Field, F. (2011) *The Foundation Years: Preventing Poor Children Becoming Poor Adults*. London: UK Government.

Fox Harding, L. (1997) *Perspectives in Child Care Policy*. London: Longman.

Gambrill, E. (1994) What's in a name? Task centred, empirical, and behavioural practice. *Social Service Review* 68(4), 578–599.

General Social Care Council (2008) *Roles and Tasks of Social Work*. London: General Social Care Council.

Grant, L. and Kinman, G. (2014) *Developing Resilience for Social Work Practice*. Basingstoke: Palgrave.

Halmos, P. (1965) *The Faith of the Counsellors*. London: Constable.

Hanvey, C. and Philpot, T. (eds) (1994) *Practising Social Work*. London: Routledge.

Hastings, A., Bailey, N., Bramley, G. and Gannon, M. (2015) *The Cost of the Cuts: The Impact on Local Government and Poorer Communities*. York: Joseph Rowntree.

Howe, D., Brandon, M., Hinings, D. and Schofield, G. (1999) *Attachment Theory, Child Maltreatment and Family Support: A Practice and Assessment Model*. London: Palgrave.

Johnstone, R. (2016) *CIPFA Survey: Council CFOs Highlight Social Care Pressures*. Available from: www.publicfinance.co.uk/news/2016/12/cipfa-survey-council-cfos-highlight-social-care-pressures [accessed 6 February 2017].

Jones, R. (2014) *The Story of Baby P: Setting the Record Straight*. Bristol: Policy Press.

Munro, E. (2004) The impact of audit on social work practice. *British Journal of Social Work* 34, 1077–1097.

Munro, E. (2010) *The Munro Review of Child Protection Part One: A Systems Analysis*. London: The Stationery Office.

Munro, E. (2011a) *Munro Review of Child Protection: Interim Report – The Child's Journey*. London: The Stationery Office.

Munro, E. (2011b) *The Munro Review of Child Protection: Final Report, a Child-Centred System*. London: The Stationery Office.

Munro, E. (2012) *Progress Report: Moving Towards a Child Centred System*. London: The Stationery Office.

Murphy, M. (2004) *Developing Collaborative Relationships in Interagency Child Protection Work*. Lyme Regis: Russell House Publishing.

Narey, M. (2014) *Making the Education of Social Workers Consistently Effective*. London: Stationery Office.

Norgrove, D. (2011) *Family Justice Review Final Report*. London: UK Government.

Parton, N. (2016) The contemporary politics of child protection: part two (The BASPCAN Founders Lecture 2015). *Child Abuse Review* 25(1), 9–16.

Payne, M. (2006) *What is Professional Social Work*. Bristol: Policy Press.

Payne, M. (2014) *Modern Social Work Theory* (4th edn). Basingstoke: Palgrave Macmillan.

Ruch, G. (2013) Understanding contemporary social work: we need to talk about relationships. In Parker, J. and Doel, M. (eds) *Professional Social Work*. London: SAGE.

Scott, S., Sylva, K., Beckett, C., Kallitsoglou, A., Doolan, M. and Ford, T. (2012) Should parenting programmes to improve children's life chances address child behaviour, reading skills, or both? Rationale for the Helping Children Achieve trial. *European Journal Of Developmental Psychology* 9(1), 47–60.

Seebohm, F. (chair) (1968) *Report of the Committee on Local Authority and Allied Social Services*. London: The Stationery Office.

Sheldon, B. (1978) Theory & practice in social work: a re-examination of a tenuous relationship. *British Journal of Social Work* 8(1), 1–22.

Tickell, C. (2011) *The Early Years: Foundations for Life, Health and Learning*. London: UK Government.

Tobis, D. (2013) *From Pariahs to Partners: How Parents and Their Allies Changed New York City's Child Welfare System*. Oxford: Oxford University Press.

Tunstill, J., Aldgate, J. and Hughes, M. (2006) *Improving Children's Service Networks*. London: Jessica Kingsley Press.

Turnell, A. and Edwards, S. (1999) *Signs of Safety: A Safety and Solution Oriented Approach to Child Protection Casework*. New York: WW Norton.

TrussellTrust (2012) *Foodbank Statistics*. Available from: www.trusselltrust.org/news-a nd-blog/latest-stats/end-year-stats/#fy-2011-2012 [accessed on 6 February 2017].

Webber, M., Reidy, H., Ansari, D., Stevens, M. and Morris, D. (2015) Enhancing social networks: a qualitative study of health and social care practice in UK mental health services. *Health and Social Care in the Community* 23, 180–189.

Wilkins, D. and Boahen, G. (2013) *Critical Analysis Skills for Social Workers*. London: McGraw Hill.

PART I

Practice near research

3

DIFFICULT CONVERSATIONS ON THE FRONT LINE

Observations of home visits to talk about neglect

Fiona Henderson

This chapter takes the reader on a journey through a research study I conducted looking at face-to-face communication in child protection social work. I describe the way in which my curiosities and hunches about social work practice became the starting point for a qualitative study using observation and interview techniques informed by psychoanalysis. As a psychotherapist, I became interested in how social work feels on the front line and how psychoanalytic ideas can help make sense of the everyday difficulties of the social worker's task. The exploratory phase of the study led me to focus on the tensions arising from social workers' shared responsibilities for care and control, and how these tensions affect conversations with parents when there are serious concerns about neglect. By showing how the research process unfolds, I hope to encourage other practitioners to follow up their questions in a similar way, by designing studies which can shed light on the challenges of the difficult work we do.

Phase 1: Getting inspired

Several years ago the BBC ran a documentary series called *Protecting our Children* (BBC2, January 2012) which followed in detail the work of a children and families social work team in Bristol. This television series was credited with being the first sensitive and accurate exposure of child protection social work ever screened in the UK, helping to challenge judgemental attitudes that were common at the time. It sparked in me a wish to conduct a practice-near-research study into social work as it takes place in the real setting of family homes.

Watching the programmes, I felt extremely moved by the predicament of these practitioners who we saw entering the squalid, bewildering and frightening homes of very disturbed, young parents. I was struck by the distractions and anxieties that filled these fraught encounters, and by the observations and conversations upon which enormous decisions had to be based about the safety of children. It seemed like doing finely tuned work in the midst of a war zone.

In one programme, a newly qualified social worker visits her first family by herself. The parents are fractious and intimidating and the skin on the social worker's neck flushes red with anxiety as she sits in midst of their onslaught. This was agonisingly difficult work in horrific conditions and with the weight of public opinion bearing down on her, not to mention the television cameras.

In another case, a more experienced social worker had a decision to make about the safety of an unborn child of two unstable, adolescent parents. We watched her become rapidly and prematurely hopeful, even excited, when the pregnant mother announced that she'd broken off her relationship with the father who was clearly a very agitated young man. The social worker's euphoria crashed and she broke down in tears soon after, when the young mother ran away to rejoin the father, abandoning her newborn baby in the foster home. This social worker had to leave her job for a while due to stress.

These practitioners were courageous in exposing their work, and their emotional responses to the work. But it also struck me how personally exposed they were to the effects of the clients' disturbance because they lacked a theoretical framework to help them think about what they were encountering. For example, the sudden, elated optimism evoked by the pregnant woman was strongly suggestive of a manic defence involving denial and splitting rather than healthy insight on the mother's part. If the social worker had been able to recognise this at the time, she might have realised that the apparent change was, in fact, highly precarious.

Watching these programmes, it struck me that psychoanalytic ideas could help social workers make better sense of what is going on when they are with their clients. Concepts such as transference, countertransference and projective identification offer ways of understanding what happens beneath the surface of conversations – the pushes and pulls of communication – which can throw practitioners off course and make the work feel confusing and difficult. Social workers are very observant about their clients, but without theory to apply to their observations they are vulnerable to being disturbed and overwhelmed themselves.

Phase 2: Reflecting on my own practice

For many years I worked alongside social workers in an assessment team for families involved in care proceedings. It often seemed that my social work colleagues had a more complicated relationship with the parents because of their statutory role. As a psychotherapist, I had more freedom to get to know parents in depth and to risk being unpopular when sensitive matters were brought up. I thought there was something particular about social work which stirred conflicts and tensions, and affected communication in subtle but important ways.

Social workers wear the two hats of care professional and agent of the law. They have to build relationships with clients around agreed, and often unrealistic, goals, while also monitoring them on behalf of the state, with powers to instigate legal processes which can alter the course of a family's life for good. This situation can be contradictory and uncomfortable for practitioners, who feel that caring is the reason they came into the work and control is a burden they would rather not carry. It can be hard to exercise authority if we associate it with coercion and other forms of unwelcome force, and we can lose sight of more therapeutic notions of authority like challenging, limit-setting and saying 'no'. Social workers told me how building relationships with clients can seem like a luxury they never have, when home visits are nearly always to raise difficult matters: 'It's tough to be so unpopular; just seeing our telephone numbers coming up on their phones is enough.' Clients often harbour traumatic recollections of social workers from childhoods spent in local authority care. Feelings connected with such trauma are often projected into practitioners who come to represent all that is neglectful and abusive from their past. When these children become parents themselves it seems inevitable that their engagement will be jaundiced if painful memories are reawakened by social workers being on the scene again.

It can be hard to be clear and truthful about care and control when working with reluctant clients. We might be tempted to deny or minimise one role in order to emphasise the other; for example, teaming up with a client sympathetically and talking about statutory procedures and expectations as if they belong somewhere else. In this way, our authority is split off and projected into 'the system', which can then be seen as 'cruel', leaving us free for a collusive alliance of sorts: a rather disingenuous version of 'care'.

Social workers might also feel driven to exaggerate their custodial role, becoming authoritarian and harsh, and out of touch with the client's struggle. There might be pressure to achieve compliance with 'agreed' goals despite the client's obvious resistance or distress. Social workers can worry that if they become 'too soft' this will be exploited by clients and efforts towards change will not be made.

With the emphasis on partnership in social work, we need a better understanding of how partnership with clients can be sustained while painful realities are faced. Psychoanalytic ideas about ambivalent states of mind can be useful here – talking to clients about their wish to reject the very help and support they also crave. These theories have shown the importance of facing honestly with clients the limitations of what can be offered and what can be achieved, for example, talking with a client about how troubled they still feel at the end of an intervention where small but important gains have also been made. It can be helpful if the social worker conveys that they too can bear feelings of guilt and sadness about this situation.

Social workers can feel so driven to achieve goals that they shield parents from ordinary responsibilities like attending appointments on time or getting their children to school. We can be quick to book taxis or escort parents to meetings to make sure that they turn up. At the same time we are trying to help parents take a more mature approach to their children's needs. This conflict between ensuring and enabling change can send ambiguous messages to parents about what is expected of them, and can play into tensions, often unconscious, between infantile and adult aspects of their functioning.

In child protection work our language can become defensive if we shy away from spelling out uncomfortable truths. It can be hard to gauge our true level of concern if we use muted terms and clichés in order not to frighten the client away. For example, poor parenting is often described as 'not meeting your child's needs', serious problems in a child as 'significant harm' and meeting other parents as 'accessing relationships'. This way of talking is picked up by clients too and can lead to a collusive avoidance of frankness, as if serious matters can't be faced. In a similar way, social workers described the usefulness of texting to reach clients in a less intrusive way. But there is also the possibility that texts might be used defensively to avoid a more direct conversation about something difficult.

Social workers have to grapple with tensions between paternalism and partnership all the time to help them make authoritative interventions in a therapeutic way. Part of this process involves reflecting on one's own relationship to power and authority based on past experiences of key figures in our lives. In my research I wanted to understand how these tensions affect everyday practice and I was surprised to find that there were few existing studies of real conversations between social workers and clients, with most relying on hypothetical case vignettes or actors (Forrester et al., 2007; Forrester et al., 2008) or retrospective accounts of interviews based on social workers' memory (Thoburn et al., 1995). We know much less about what happens during real encounters in clients' homes, particularly the dynamics of face-to-face interviews, when tension between care and control can be very close to the surface.

Phase 3: Observations from a pilot study

My study took place in the real setting of a local authority child and family team and involved ongoing cases where there were significant concerns about neglect. To familiarise myself with how the team worked I attended professionals' meetings in an observing role. I was particularly interested in whether tensions in social workers between care and control could be noticed during their interviews with clients and, if so, what effect these tensions might be having on the interaction going on. Below are two excerpts from these meetings; identifying details have been changed and my commentary is in square brackets.

First observation

This was an interview between a social worker (SW) and a parent (P) during a professionals' meeting. The professionals talk amongst themselves in a circle with P sitting silently amongst them. Their focus is on the precise wording of the written agreement which P is being asked to sign. It is as if the written agreement is responsible for parenting P's child and not P herself, and so the wording has to be 'just right'. There also seems to be a wishful fantasy around that P's signature will guarantee her compliance, although everyone knows that this is far from the case. P then begins to complain about the professionals' interference in her life:

P: The police were called over the weekend, how come?

SW: Well, it was me who requested the welfare assessment.

[This seemed like a coded way of saying 'I called the police'.]

P: [In a patronising tone] They were running around all over the place.

SW: [More firmly] What I would need to say is … what I need to say is … we need to face some tough questions … that need to be asked … Questions like … We need to ask what alternative carers might be available who could look after C?

[P seems full of fury and tears but has no space to express this.]

SW: We have information from reliable sources that you were not there on Friday or Saturday evening. What happened that you were in a position where you were unable to care for C over the weekend?

[P starts crying; tension rises in the room.]

SW: Would you like to take a break?

P: No, I'm OK.

TEACHER: Where were you over the weekend?

[P gives a plausible story; there is relief in the room.]

SW: [Trying to soften the tone] What's making it difficult to be at home?

[Tension rises again; P becomes rambling and verbose, seemingly as a way of settling herself down; tension in the room eases.]

SW: [Trying to cut through P's flow] We don't need to be concerned about these other issues right now.

[SW then resumes a serious discussion of the local authority's concerns; P cries more despairingly.]

SW: Shall we take a break? Let's get some tissues.

[SW leaves the room.]

SW had a naturally empathic manner and she was also able to speak quite firmly to P about the concerns. However, on two occasions, P became upset or annoyed which made SW anxious and led her to become more concrete and solicitous, suggesting that they take a break, and leaving the room to get tissues. This kind of response seemed unnecessary for P, it interrupted the flow of the interview and an opportunity was lost for exploring P's emerging feelings more directly. P might also have felt confused by the fluctuation in the social worker's approach, towards and away from frank discussion. I thought that the social worker became anxious that she had harmed P, or her positive link with P, by confronting her with things that P didn't want to hear but needed to consider. This anxiety led the social worker to collapse the frame of the interview (by suggesting they take a break) at just the point when P became more openly distressed, a sign that she was grappling with the issues. We can hypothesise that this collapse is also experienced by P, unconsciously, as a repetition of previous failures of containment in her early life, a clue to understanding her emotional situation more fully.

Second observation

This was an interview between another social worker (SW) and a parent (M) during a professionals' meeting. M is the mother of an anorexic girl (X) who is emotionally unstable and using recreational drugs. Teacher (T).

M: I think X has lots of fears, lots of things she's worried about, so won't losing control with drugs make it worse? Your report has been in my kitchen for three weeks. She's only just looked at it this morning. She doesn't like the way she's been described as attention seeking.

[There is an atmosphere of hopelessness and despair in the room.]

M: If I told her half the things we've discussed here I think it would crush her. How long do we have to continue without telling her the truth?

SW: What can we physically do as social care? Probably not a lot; perhaps the police …

[SW returns to the care plan as the agenda and invites a psychologist to give a summary of her work with X. The psychologist says that X talked about turning 16 soon and is planning to leave home, calling it 'my way out'; M's sadness about this is obvious.]

M: And yet, when we suggested an apprenticeship, we spoke to her about visiting the college and she wasn't interested. She throws all her anger at me. If people don't get to the truth about what's really going on for her we'll never make progress.

[SW returns to the care plan; it seems as though M's sadness can't be approached; a school teacher talks about how the school feels that X has 'missed the boat' and the parents should withdraw her to avoid being prosecuted for X's non-attendance. There is a feeling around the table of agencies pulling away from X and her family.]

SW: She can actually leave home once she's 16. From our protocols if a 16 year old presents as homeless then we would have a duty to assess whether she was intentionally homeless.

[SW goes on talking about safeguarding plans, child protection plans, child in need plans; it sounds like background noise of procedural jargon, detached from the person in question, X.]

SW: There really are limitations as to what we can and cannot do. I have had a conversation with X about her situation … we would have a duty to see that she was not on the streets.

M: [Becoming more desperate] So how does her eating disorder impact on all of this? The other day I checked her weight and it was 49 kilos. I had to try and get her to eat a proper meal. Now what would have happened if I hadn't done that?

SW: If you weren't around then … she's lucky that you are around … but realistically she will end up … in hospital. I think this feels really uncomfortable for all of us here, and for you.

[This feels like a helpful, caring response which enables M to say more.]

M: She has no concern for herself at all, she just doesn't care. As soon as I go out the room she hides her food.

SW: I think that's something we drew up in the written agreement that X did sign. That as a minimum she will eat a proper meal once a day and let you check her weight. Does she do this? And that she will attend her medical appointments. One positive is that she is coming home in the evenings.

[This feels like SW pulling back from care and moving into control.]

M: Yes, but as soon as she turns 16 …

SW: The situation hasn't changed much at all apart from the positive that the police haven't been called at all since last meeting, and that's a bonus in terms of safeguarding issues.

[False optimism in the face of despair.]

SW: [Rather impatiently] So what can we do? I mean, I think clearly school is not an option for her any more.

M: I just wonder what signal it will send to X if we withdraw her from school.

T: Many children drop out of school and pick up their education later.

M: If we unroll her from school then we're letting her down.

SW: Can I just return to the plan? If the day unit is involved they can inform her about her options and choices but unless she wants to follow through it won't make any difference.

T: But I think you want to demonstrate to X that you still care as a parent.

SW: I think if you remove the eating disorder then we might not be sitting round this table. We see so many teenagers with similar issues.

M: X wants me when she's down and hates me when she's all worked up.

T: I think things feel just a bit better than when we last met.

SW: [Eagerly] Yes, I have a few ticks on my form here.

T: Are you getting support yourself [to M]?

SW: We discussed this last time ... I think we've got to be realistic ... We do have to bear in mind that, at 16, she might say 'I'm not staying at home'. The police are still on the plan, even after that. After X's birthday ... I'll come and see her and ask what her intentions are ... if we could plan ... Let's meet after her birthday and then we can see, is she going to leave home and turn up somewhere. Meanwhile, I'll come out and see X.

In this interview, the social worker appeared anxious about the extent of M's demands and needs, so much so that she became managerial and controlling in an effort to keep M's feelings at bay. The social worker came across as emotionally detached from the emerging material, which prevented her being properly available to listen to M and discover what might be going on. She seemed to feel compelled to drive through an outcome in the form of a care plan and to limit any expectations on herself, or her organisation, which could be regarded as 'unreasonable'.

There is a key moment in the exchange when the social worker makes an empathic remark which seems, momentarily, to deepen emotional contact with M. I thought that the social worker sensed this emotional contact and pulled back from it, quite rapidly, by becoming more controlling, talking about the agenda and care plan. This can be understood as a defensive retreat by the social worker in response to the client's projection of helplessness and despair. At times, the social worker's need to avoid and control was picked up by others in the meeting, who then tried to offer an empathic and caring response themselves.

A brief reflective discussion with the social worker afterwards explored how she found the meeting with M:

FH: How do you feel after the meeting?

SW: Relief that I survived it.

[There is a sense of SW's bravado in the face of sadness and despair. SW is also very keen to get feedback from me.]

SW: How was I?

FH: How do you think it went?

SW: OK considering. We've come some way from last time when we didn't have a plan; we were just a group of professionals and a girl, a young woman, who was all over the place. Now at least we've come together and can share the responsibility for how chaotic and risky she is. We each know what everyone else is doing and that, even though she doesn't want to engage, there are bits of ... some of us ... she is seeing regularly. The main thing is sharing responsibility for the risk ... and the fact that she's making an informed consent not to do things like school.

FH: What felt hard in the meeting?

SW: [Pausing to reflect] The way Mum kept going on about X's schooling all the time. It is hard, she's bound to be really worried.

FH: I thought there was an atmosphere of sadness and despair in the room.

SW: [Slightly defensively] Well yes, definitely, we all feel despair about the fact that she won't engage with help.

FH: I wonder if, when it feels so hopeless, you feel like you have to be more active, get the group working on the plan; like you have to keep the group buoyed up, the only oxygen in the room?

SW: Well yes, I do try and bring the focus back to the plan. [She laughs at the thought of being 'the oxygen']

In this reflective discussion the social worker reveals her considerable anxiety that she will be isolated in the work and overwhelmed by the risks and demands of the case. She allows herself a brief moment of empathy for the client when she says 'It's hard, she's bound to be really worried'. When I respond by describing the 'atmosphere of sadness and despair' she retreats from her earlier caring stance and speaks in a more formulaic way about the shared despair of the group. The social worker had difficulty using my observation to help her reflect on her work. I thought she felt exposed by my presence and anxious about how I might be judging her. This rapid oscillation towards and then away from empathy with the client during our discussion mirrored a similar movement that occurred in the interview itself.

This exploratory phase of my research allowed me to see how social workers use good communication skills to combine their care and risk management roles. Their frank and practical approach helps them to be open with clients about difficult matters but they are still affected in subtle ways by aspects of clients' emotional lives which make them anxious or which they struggle to understand. During the interviews there were times when the social workers seemed to avoid or turn away from emotional contact with the parent. This struck me as important and I decided to make these deviations the main focus of my study and to investigate whether, as I suspected, they were connected to increased tension between care and control.

Phase 4: The main study

My study tested the prediction that there are moments during interviews with parents when significant, and largely unconscious, tension can arise for social workers because care and control cannot be reconciled. At these times social workers can find themselves deviating from their core task in unintended and avoidant ways. These diversions, or 'moments of avoidance' (MOAs), act as an unconscious defence for social worker and client, distracting them from something that is unapproachable at that particular time. I wanted to investigate whether these moments of avoidance could be found in everyday practice, and if so, why they might be occurring at these particular times.

To collect my data, I joined social workers on their home visits in a mainly silent, observing role, travelling with them in their cars to gain an impression of the anxieties that these visits evoked. I wrote detailed 'process recordings' immediately afterwards from memory, setting out a moment-by-moment account of the dialogue, action and interpersonal dynamics between the social worker and parent, and paying close attention to areas where the social worker seemed to avoid or move away from something that was going on. I also made notes about the emotional atmosphere of interview and any spontaneous thoughts and feelings I had while I was there; this was a way to pick up unconscious tensions that might be stirring during the encounter.

The process recordings were analysed for the presence or absence of MOAs using a brief schedule of defining features such as tone, deviation and emotional distance. The analysis was 'triangulated' by presenting it to other researchers so that I could gain distance from the immediacy of the experience and be open to new perspectives on my data.

Key findings

It was possible to identify brief MOAs during interviews with parents according to a number of recognisable features. At these times the social worker would be diverted or distracted away from areas of emotional tension into a more comfortable way of talking. Some diversions seemed to be deliberate, tactful responses to the client's distress, while other avoidance seemed unconscious and based on heightened tension in the social worker at the time. I made this distinction by attending to my intuitive responses at the time and later, when analysing the data, and when stepping back from the material on several occasions to discuss my findings with others.

This is a disguised excerpt from my process recording of Case A – observation of an interview between social worker 'Mark' and a mother of three children 'Tina'. The case has been open since the children's birth due to concerns about neglect. The children have come and gone from foster care but the concerns remain, alongside short periods of improvement. Currently, poor school attendance and Tina's frequent 'disappearances' are the main issues. The case is heading towards a child protection conference and Tina is very upset with Mark about this.

The social worker describes the aim of this visit as being 'to get Tina to see that, as agreed, she must get the children to school on time or else … we'll have to go back to conference'. On the way, he says 'I feel heavy-hearted, anticipating having the same conversation I've had a million times and waiting to see what kinds of excuses and manoeuvres she will try this time'. We can hear how his initial 'tough talk' quickly gives way to despair, as he feels caught up in a cynical, cat-and-mouse routine with the client that is hard to bring out into the open with her in a straightforward way.

My commentary on the psychoanalytic process of the interview is included in straight text and highlights two identified MOAs (**[MOA1]** and **[MOA2]**). I thought that both MOAs occurred as a response to tension in the social worker between care and control which I was able to pick up at the time.

MARK: Well Tina, today we have to have a conversation about what's in the written agreement and mainly about the children's school attendance. School tell me this past week K's attendance has been only 37%.

Mark gets straight to the point, asserting himself clearly in his risk-monitoring role.

TINA: Really? How come? That can't be right … I mean he's had a really bad cold. In fact, ever since January we seem to have been ill, I don't know why.

M: It's not just bad, it's really bad Tina, way not good enough and it has to improve. The school still tell me that they can't get hold of you and that you're not keeping them informed about why the children are not in. You've said that K's been ill but all you have to do, Tina, is call them, it's not my job to do that for you, this is your responsibility. I can't keep tags all the time on whether they're in school and this figure is atrocious.

Mark is not deterred by Tina's earlier evasiveness and he spells out the concerns very firmly, using her own word 'bad' to highlight her minimisation. He uses Tina's name to link up with her while he confronts her with difficult matters, skilfully combining care and control. His use of the strong adjective 'atrocious' conveys a capacity to face facts truthfully and robustly.

T: How can it be 37%? We were off Thursday and then Monday was a holiday too, then he was ill on Tuesday.

Tina is uncomfortable and defensive and responds to Mark's confrontation by stalling for time, presenting extraneous, concrete details and creating a diversion. She may experience Mark in a persecutory way at that particular moment or she may simply feel caught out.

M: **[MOA1]** The percentage gets worked out on a weekly basis and last week was a 4 day week and K only went in 2 days so that adds up to 50% and then that gets balanced with the previous week where K's attendance was 42% and so … [he sighs]. If they're ill then it's a simple matter of picking up the phone and letting school know.

Seemingly in response to Tina's diversion, Mark falls into a moment of avoidance **[MOA1]** where he too becomes concrete and taken up with fine details.

However, with his sigh he catches himself and recovers his authority by spelling out what needs to happen. He knows the children are rarely ill and that their absence from school is more complicated than this. Mark conveys a note of despair as he meets Tina's resistance, yet again. The moment of avoidance seems to stem from anxiety that his previous remark was too harsh. At this moment Mark may be struggling, unconsciously, with a conflict between care and control.

T: Doctor's note ... they have a new system at the school of just recording it as illness and ... Oh Mark, you must think I'm a nightmare. I do need to work on the things that need sorting out. There's also been a lot of allegations of P dealing drugs at school and it would be good to get that sorted out once and for all. [Becoming imploring] Honestly, I do believe her.

Tina tries to continue her avoidance through pedantic, concrete talk about the school system, but she senses that Mark is not 'buying it' this time, as conveyed by his stillness and his fixed expression. She appeals to Mark directly, by name, which has the effect of disarming him. She then turns to talking about her daughter P as a new focus of concern, and this distracts Mark's attention away from her.

M: **[MOA2]** Well there is a project where young people can take a 40-day challenge if there are these kind of allegations, to clear their name. Do you think P would be prepared to do that?

Mark is swayed by Tina's diversion into focussing on what P needs to do, and away from Tina's own responsibilities as a parent. However it is complicated because he is required to prioritise the needs of a child at all times. Mark is momentarily thrown by Tina's direct appeal to him by name, and again, he falls in line with her diversion on to her child. This was a momentary collusion with Tina's defence while at the same time he conveyed firmness through his physical posture.

T: [Sounding relieved] Yes, I hope so? Drug testing would be the best thing.

Tina is 'off-the-hook' and regains control of the interview again by talking prescriptively about her child. Her relief suggests that her diversion was a defensive manoeuvre in order to relieve tension in the room.

M: What do you think they use?
T: Weed

Mark is still caught up in the diversion with Tina, becoming sidelined into concrete discussion of P's use of drugs. Mark also has a responsibility to gather information about P's welfare and this can create a conflict during interviews where the focus and emotional impact of the discussion is lost.

In this excerpt I thought there was evidence of two MOAs where the social worker gets diverted from emotional tensions in the interview into a discussion which is more concrete and detached. A kind of 'enactment' ensues due to the unconscious effects of projective identification where the social worker falls in line with the client's projections and stops being able to think. The client offers excuses, or mentions something concerning about her child as a kind of defence, and the social worker gets distracted for a moment, away from talking about the client's responsibilities as a parent, into discussing these other issues instead.

After the home visit the social worker spoke of his frustration:

M: I keep repeating the same conversations. In some ways it's more difficult because she acknowledges it all but the results don't show. She often says 'I'm a bad mum aren't I? I'm a real "div"'. I don't know if I'm being cynical but I wonder if it's part of her act, to be disarming. Cos she's beating herself up, it's her way of not taking responsibility, cos I've heard it so many times before.

The social worker asks whether the client needs to act upon him, by talking in a self-pitying way, in order to evade guilt and responsibility that would actually be helpful for her to feel. He is aware of how powerfully and directly this way of talking can distract him, or 'win him over', and he wonders whether the client is aware of this too. The social worker's brief MOAs at these times may have been linked, unconsciously, to irritation at feeling controlled. This made it hard for him to recognise and talk about what was going on so that he and the client could think about it together.

The presence of MOAs also raises a question about whether social workers lose the focus of difficult conversations with parents because of constant pressure to check up on facts and gather new information, or because of the overriding need to prioritise the child. The challenge is to be alert to the pushes and pulls that occur during any conversation and to ask ourselves regularly '*What does it feel like right now, talking to this client?*' or '*what use is the client making of me at this particular moment? – is it to help her explore and understand, or to help her avoid or deny?*' This is not at all easy, and we may think we have more control over the direction an interview is taking than we actually do because we underestimate the powerful unconscious processes that are at work.

The psychoanalyst Betty Joseph described how patients with severe emotional instability use the analyst for their own purposes to help them with their anxiety, transforming the analysis into a 'scene for action rather than understanding' and distorting their view of the analyst and the help that is on offer (Joseph, 1978: 224). In this situation the patient will actively try to encourage the analyst to collude with their defences, to carry unwanted parts of their internal world and to act out with them in the transference. These mainly unconscious processes are mobilised to keep unbearable thoughts and feelings at bay.

In the same way, adult clients with similar difficulties use unconscious defences like splitting and projective identification to manage the intense anxiety evoked by our involvement in their lives. In my study, I saw how splitting and projection would occur, suddenly and unexpectedly, in response to something the social worker said, or when the client felt particularly anxious, under pressure, or exposed. These defences could result in an MOA by the social worker, throwing them off course, and steering them away from something difficult that should be discussed. This distraction in our work can be very frustrating, and we can literally feel 'taken for a ride' in ways that we can't make sense of at the time.

My study suggests that most MOAs take the form of an enactment – or unconscious 'dance' – where the social worker moves in the direction of more pronounced control, becoming procedural and emotionally detached, or into a placatory or collusive form of care, where social worker and client get caught up in something other than the concerns in front of them.

MOAs occurred at points where the client's emotional struggle was communicated more directly in a way which made the social worker anxious or uncomfortable, although they may not have registered this consciously at the time. Under sway of these kinds of projections, without realising, we can feel tempted to retaliate by exercising control in a harsh or unwarranted way. For example, on a home visit to a mother who was passively hostile and evasive, a social worker felt constrained, not helped by the presence of a male 'friend' who had been (un)invited round. The social worker (SW) spoke to me (FH) about it afterwards:

SW: It wasn't that easy with him chipping in all the time. If it was just me and her it would have been a different conversation. I kept thinking 'hey I'm not talking to you', but then again I was interested in his views. It was clear how he was protecting her at every move, always piping up to cover her or back her up.

FH: And this makes your job harder does it?

SW: Yes, having someone there so that I won't go too deep into a conversation so she cries ... but then again she often cries and cries. She does that such a lot ... So it's kind of like ... so then, it's easy to not focus on the children. So you've got to keep on ... keep on ... you have to be mindful of what you're there for ... Cos I think she's very good at moving the conversation away from what you're there for ... towards her ailments, her issues. It's a ploy on her part, deliberately, to avoid having a more serious talk about the children. You almost have to have a clear goal of what you're going there for, before you go, and then try and stick to it. I would have welcomed the chance to go in there with some big news about what we know, to shock her.

FH: Why is that? It's unusual to speak about wanting to shock someone.

SW: Yes, but I would have liked to have some different news to bring because ... she always minimises or normalises the situation, or acts as if you're telling her off and then going into baby mode so that you feel bad when all you're doing is trying to discuss the issues about the children ... I could have seen if it made a difference if I'd had something big to say.

FH: As if you feel it would jolt her into taking things more seriously.

SW: Yes, she works on appearing to be open, appearing to be signed up to the things you ask her, but it's false, it's just put on for you. The more she feels she gives you, the less she thinks you feel she's got something to hide. As if I'm thinking 'well, she's open and honest, that's all fine'.

FH: But you're saying it's a sham?

SW: I'm dubious. I just feel there's more to her, something she's holding back.

In this case the social worker felt provoked by the client involving a 'bouncer' friend in a way which restricted the interview. She was also irritated by the client minimising serious issues and diverting attention on to her to avoid addressing the concerns about her children. In frustration, the social worker had a fantasy of breaking through the client's defence by revealing what she knows, hoping this might shock the client out of her avoidance. Of course it is necessary to speak boldly at times but I think this social worker was worried that any such boldness would be dangerous or unkind and so she held back. Perhaps she had an inkling that her wish to confront the client was partly a wish to retaliate.

The social worker easily recognised the client's avoidance but didn't have a way of understanding its unconscious effects on her. This mother splits off her hostility and projects it into her 'friend' who is recruited to 'keep out' unwanted intrusions, rather like a menacing dog. The friend then acts out the client's hostility by intimidating the social worker and disrupting the interview. In turn, the client adopts a childish, naive persona, as if to deny her maturity and prevent anyone having ordinary adult expectations of her. The social worker feels at the mercy of these defensive manoeuvres, which she probably regards as more deliberate than they actually are. Keeping in mind concepts like splitting and projection can help us to navigate with clients when we are being buffeted around in this sort of way. The key to being alert to these processes is to keep asking ourselves how we feel in the presence of the client, even if the answer seems surprising or unacceptable to us. For example, we may feel bored and unmoved by the client's plight and this may be a response to projections of denial in a client who is unable to face the seriousness of their situation.

Conclusion

My research looked in detail at the uncomfortable moments we all recognise in our conversations with troubled parents. It highlighted the sudden and unexpected quality of unconscious projections by clients when there is heightened tension or pressure around. These projections can destabilise our thinking and perception, and can lead us into defensive exchanges with clients which detract from the important discussions we set out to have. Waddell described how in conversations with resistant families:

Words were thought to be objects, usually weapons; speaking itself became action; meaning was distorted and links systematically scrambled, lest the family's pain, and the suffering of each individual, be experienced.

(Waddell, 1989: 31)

Families who rely on primitive defences like splitting and denial can powerfully convert a thoughtful conversation into what feels, to them, like a concrete attack on their very being. They can become preoccupied with battling the help and helpers they desperately need, getting caught up in ambivalence and conflict in their dealings with us. It can be useful to have ways of talking to clients about this; for example referring to '*a part of them that wants to move forward while another part feels the risk is too great*'. This gives permission to feel hostile and reluctant about working with us alongside anxiety and hope for something better. If clients can experience us as understanding the complexities of engagement, how hard it can be to make the smallest shift towards insight and change, then they can begin to build a relationship with us which can support them through the inevitable turbulence of the work.

My aim has been to address how we manage the tensions of conflicted relationships in our safeguarding work with parents: being the caring 'good object' and the controlling 'bad object' at one and the same time. I think we can afford to be bolder in the way we confront difficult issues with parents because being firm about painful facts is not the same as being uncaring. Adults with marked personality disturbance are some of the most challenging people we meet in our work. They usually have widespread problems with relationships and day-to-day life but can be desperate not to acknowledge or address these problems and their feelings about them. They may be very skilled at avoidance and we may inadvertently reinforce this situation by colluding with historical silences around sensitive matters.

I started with a hunch that the dual responsibilities for care and control proved so irreconcilable for social workers, at times, that they found themselves retreating from emotional contact with clients into something more avoidant and defensive. Having had a closer look at real practice in home settings, I now think that this was not the whole story. The clients themselves bring emotional disturbance which influences us through powerful projections involving splitting and denial. Without ways of understanding what is happening at these moments, or afterwards in supervision, we are more vulnerable to identification with these projections and to missing something important about the family's situation. It is helpful to have strategies to keep us engaged with the purpose of the visit but to also be mindful of when these strategies can become defensive, shutting down our emotional availability and openness to the 'unthought known' (Bollas, 1987). Becoming more sensitive to the subtleties of avoidance and resistance in ourselves, and our clients, can help us work more effectively with families to support change.

Editors' afterword

Social work agencies expect social workers to make big changes in a short period of time. Usually this is unrealistic. In fact most of us know this from our experience of ourselves. Fiona's social workers seem to be attempting to make changes by going through the child protection plan. This is like trying to make a pig fatter by weighing it. In fact social workers do have one invaluable resource – themselves.

Many if not most social work clients have not had the experience of an adult taking a sustained interest in them. This is more effective if they are offered a regular day and time. This gives them some feeling of control as well as a sense that their social worker has space for them in their mind. It is important to be aware of small but significant changes. I had a female patient who was psychotic. She thought I was a man. One day she said 'I know I only *think* you are a man.'

Social workers often underestimate how important they are to a client. The significance to clients of missed appointments or even a social worker leaving is minimised. One way in which leaving is minimised is by bringing the new worker. This puts an unreasonable demand on the client to be polite to someone they do not know while not being allowed to say goodbye to their usual worker. Farewells can be a complex process, and an opportunity to do a small piece of work. A social worker brought the new social worker to visit a client she had known for some time. As they left the client said to the new worker 'I don't think I will remember your name.' The client is feeling unwanted and projects this experience on to the new worker.

References

Bollas, C. (1987) *The Shadow of the Object: Psychoanalysis of the Unthought Known*. London: Free Association Books.

Forrester, D., McCambridge, J., Waissbein, C. and Rollnick, S. (2007) How do child and family social workers talk to parents about child welfare concerns? *Child Abuse Review* 16, 1–13.

Forrester, D., Kershaw, S., Moss, H. and Hughes, L. (2008) Communication skills in child protection: how do social workers talk to parents? *Child & Family Social Work* 13, 41–51.

Joseph, B. (1978) Different types of anxiety and their handling in the analytic situation. *International Journal of Psychoanalysis* 59, 223–228.

Thoburn, J., Lewis, A. and Shemmings, D. (1995) *Paternalism or Partnership? Family Involvement in the Child Protection Process*. London: The Stationery Office.

Waddell, M. (1989) Living in two worlds: psychodynamic theory and social work practice. *Free Associations* 15, 11–35.

4

WRITTEN ON THE BODY

Charlotte Noyes

Introduction

This chapter originated from a doctoral research project, which explored the impact of direct work on social work practitioners in the field of statutory child and family work. The choice of this research topic was determined by my desire, as a social worker with over 25 years experience in this field, to go below the surface and examine how social workers went about undertaking their primary task and to explore lived day-to-day social work practice.

In this chapter I will present material from my research and the findings and hypotheses derived from it. The initial section will use excerpts from interviews with social work practitioners, when they talked about their experiences of their work, and then proceed to consider the meaning of this data, drawing on relevant theory. The final section will explore implications for practice.

It is not within the scope of this chapter to comment on the sociological, cultural, political or historical issues that relate to this particular area of social work practice. However, these issues are significant in locating social work with children and families in its present day context, so I would direct the reader to consult texts from Parton (1985; 1991; 2008; 2012; 2014), Ferguson (2004, 2007), Hoggett (2000), Jones (2014a, 2014b), Munro (2005, 2011a, 2011b) and Warner (2015) for background and analysis of the past and current issues for the profession.

Direct work – what is the social work experience?

That direct work has such an impact on workers is not a new concept and has been explored by others including: Mattinson (1975); Mattinson and Sinclair (1979); Preston-Shoot and Agass (1990); Bower (2005); Ruch, Turney and Ward (2010).

Mattinson and Sinclair (1979) writing in *Mate and Stalemate* detailed an action research project in statutory children and families' work and perhaps gives some of the most authentic reports of direct contact with clients and examples of just how disturbing and unsettling this can be for workers. This classic text is, in my view, essential reading for any social worker, and the 'Suckers or Bastards' chapter presents an account of how unsettling direct interaction between service users and practitioners can be. In this chapter, Mattinson and Sinclair recount an incident one Friday afternoon in which a client, a Mrs Yates, attended the office in what seemed to be a highly agitated and aroused state. She shouted and screamed and used verbal obscenities and her behaviour veered wildly from intense anger, which included acts of destruction, to extreme distress. Mrs Yates had brought her children with her and they were witness to, and involved in, the uncontrolled and apparently irrational behaviour of their mother. The incident lasted for several hours as Mrs Yates left the office and then returned, demanding money and simultaneously asking for the social workers to take her children into care and preventing them from doing just that. The incident concluded as stated by the authors:

> The area officer and I needed each other for support to withstand the fury and obstinacy with which we were confronted. In desperation I asked Mrs Yates why she had to make us behave like such bastards towards her. She screamed that we were bastards and rather wearily I agreed that maybe we were. Almost at once she began to soften and decided to leave with the children. She left us drained and shattered.
>
> *(Mattinson and Sinclair, 1979: 137–139)*

This is an excellent illustration of how powerful and disturbing the impact of direct encounters can be and how complex and multi-layered these incidents and exchanges are. It is not just the superficial agenda – Mrs Yates wanting money – but deeper and often unconscious desires and conflict that are communicated. These processes require unpicking in order to be understood and some sense made for the individual client or family.

In the research the day-to-day social work task was examined, including paying attention to the role and impact of organisational issues and dynamics. The aim was to learn more about how social workers went about their task, particularly home visits, as surprisingly given the centrality of the home visit in child and family social work, there is relatively little research into this area – the notable exception is of course Harry Ferguson's work (Ferguson 2003; 2004; 2005; 2008; 2009; 2010; 2011a; 2011b; 2013; 2014). I wanted to know more about what practitioners were actually doing and their experience of undertaking the primary task.

I identified a team – a Child in Need (CIN) team – and met with them and their managers obtaining their consent for the research. Then for approximately six months I spent time each week observing them going about the routine social work tasks – in the office, in meetings, on home visits and then interviewing them – asking specifically about their experiences of undertaking home visits.

It was the data from these interviews that I examined in detail in my thesis. I experienced what the social workers told me as profoundly moving and significant in terms of the impact direct work with children and families can have on the practitioner – emotionally and physically – and how this might be understood and made sense of.

What they said and how they said it

It was not just what the social workers talked about that was so profoundly moving, it was also the *manner* of their communication in the interviews. As they talked they appeared at times to be re-experiencing particular events or incidents and the impact of what were often deeply disturbing and troubling encounters were conveyed non-verbally, through actions, gesture, tone of voice, volume, speed and manner of the discourse. This non-verbal communication appeared to be embedded in the bodies of the practitioners and even recalling past events could elicit physical symptoms in the interviews, such that it appeared that the social workers were not just telling me about their experiences, they were also *showing* me how it had affected them – then and in the present.

What did the workers speak about in the interviews? In the main, they talked about the families and children that seemed to have the most negative impact on them and their struggle to make sense of and process these encounters. 'Mandy' (M) spoke about the home visit she had undertaken just prior to the interview as can be seen in the following extract:

CN: Okay, um, well I wanted to speak to you today because we went out on a home visit this morning, you were kind enough to let me observe a home visit. I suppose for me, and that's part of my research, is thinking with social workers about how that is for you and maybe we could start off by you saying what you thought you were going to do or you might find initially.

M: I thought that it was a new case; that I hadn't met the mother or baby, so I think that … it as always you do have a precon … I read the paperwork from the previous social worker and had created an impression that this mother was doing, fairly well. I was aware she was a young woman um and that she'd experienced difficulties in her life, emotional difficulties throughout her own parenting, which led to her self-harming as an adolescent and that she'd had, her break-up of her relationship in pregnancy, which, I was under no doubt that you know that would have quite a serious impact on her. But I was under the impression that she was coping with parenting, quite confidently, I felt, I thought that she would be managing maybe just the basic care tasks quite well. Um, it was definitely presented to me that this is a 'child in need' case, which often we shouldn't minimise because they can be just as complex as child protection cases, but, you do have that kind of 'okay, she's a young mum with a baby, but it's CIN, it's child in need, it's not going to be at child protection level'.

So I went with probably a level of um complacency that I'd meet a mum who you know would be doing okay but might be experiencing some emotional trauma and needed maybe a bit of support. What I was faced with when I arrived was something very different, which kind of, it did unsettle me; it definitely put me on the back foot, because I suppose it was trying to regroup my thoughts in a very quick, short space of time in her presence, because I was quite surprised at what I saw really. From immediately walking in and seeing sort of Tixylix, which my immediate you know … I suppose as social workers we do go in and your observation skills are immediately switched on and you know you're starting looking, particularly with young babies you want to see that they've got adequate places to sleep and it's safe as well. And so when I saw the cough medicine I did immediately begin to think you know… it was a trigger of concern, not only that it said toddler on it, and obviously checking that it was okay for a baby to have, but immediately my mind was thinking it's, it's kind of an easy solution.

Yes I suppose … I made an assumption, from the information that had been handed over, that I'd probably find it. A, more competent … not only just competent in her presentation, maybe somebody who was more (pause) … she's young, she's 21 but maybe still with a level of maturity. I kind of walked in thinking she presented as being somebody … in her in her own physical presentation and in her interactions as being much younger and I suppose, that influenced how I spoke to her and, and …

And:

M: But it being presented as this mum just needing a bit of support when, actually, she does need support but I came away feeling really concerned about a four-month old baby.

CN: Can you talk more about that, what it was that concerned you particularly?

M: She just didn't look like a well-cared for baby … I suppose that's what struck me; as I said, the minute you walk in your antenna's up, you're looking at the environment, you are really making judgements and assessments all rolled in. I walked in, I'm looking to see a baby, I want to see a baby who's in an appropriate bedding for their age, you know that they're lying in an appropriate position, obviously straight away clocked Tixylix, you check the labels always, especially with the little ones. But just when she woke up and, and mum brought her … she just … for a four-month old baby immediately my eyes were drawn to her dirty finger nails, which is an indicator because, she's not crawling. So babies who have got dirty finger nails, how do they get dirt under their nails? Her nails were all jaggedy, they weren't they hadn't been clipped but they wouldn't be breaking because she's far too … they're just unclipped, her hands were cold, you know her face looked a bit mottled, she just didn't look like a rosy pink baby whose, she didn't smell clean, or strongly of a baby-type product, she didn't smell strongly of … she didn't smell like she hadn't been washed, but that was the impression I got that she wasn't you know … her face was a little bit … there was some snot and a little bit of dirt but nothing strongly to make you think really this baby hasn't been washed or cared for in sort of four or five days, just not … It's that low level that I don't think she's woken up in the morning and given a top and tail and put in a clean suit and had a nappy change. Those sorts of things that make you think it's just a basic task, what's the routine like. But that would correlate with how mum looked, because mum obviously hadn't got up and had a bath or a wash, or maybe tied her hair back or brushed her teeth. It's those things that you think, that's that's the setting for that routine and when mum talked about her own life and how she wanted things to be different for Y, I think, she really does need to look on routines.

CN: Yes, when you were talking with her, how did that feel for you in terms of who was doing the work?

M: I felt it was me just … obviously it's really hard, … because when you have just met somebody (pause) I suppose because she wasn't … um really, it's not just assertive or forthcoming, she was quite happy to sit there. I suppose in one sense I was really pleased because she was in and I got through the door. So I,

CN: Yes and you said that beforehand, didn't you, there was a history for her not turning up for appointments and not making herself available.

M: And cancelling cancelling at the last minute saying she wasn't well, cancelling the visit, cancelling the visit. So I suppose I was really pleased that she was in and she opened the door and that was great, so. I suppose that had also given me a slight impression that she might be a … not a difficult but avoiding or not really interested and I don't understand why social workers are involved …

And:

M: But I was surprised she was … I was going to say green, she wasn't really anything, she was quite flat, she didn't either try and placate me by … she didn't over the top say 'yeah, yeah yeah I'm going to take her to the doctors' today, don't worry', to get me off her back, but she didn't either say 'get lost, mind your own business, I know what I'm doing'. She was just passive, she didn't give me a lot, that increased my concerns, as we were talking it increased my concerns, because I just thought she's somebody who could be very easily influenced by others or quite vulnerable to people who could exploit her or Y. And as that went on I thought this is becoming … more apparent, so it felt like I was you know … anything I said to her was met by a 'yes, okay', but nothing, that reassured me, made me feel confident in her parenting or just just simply taking on some advice really and acting on it.

And:

CN: What were you thinking when you were leaving about things?

M: I was thinking 'oh my goodness, four-month old baby, high risk of cot death', that's truthfully what I thought. [laughs]

CN: And you've put your hand on your chest now.

M: Yes, cot death, cot death, that's what I thought, that was my first thought. I thought cold, chest infection, cigarettes, mum's a smoker in the home, that's what I thought, that was my biggest concern, just too ... all in a high risk group all cot death, that's what I worried for. [Sighs]

And:

M: Gosh, I came back into my office, I spoke to my colleagues ... excuse me [drinks water] ... spoke to my colleagues, which I think really had an offload, came in and spoke to the principal and a couple of the other social workers in there and said [sighs] 'it's cold, it's cold'. I think I must have said it's cold, it's so cold in there several times and ... and shared with them ...

Kate

Kate (K) talked about two families, one in particular she experienced as exceptionally difficult and left her very troubled and unsettled, but she chose not to speak about this family initially and introduced another, before it seemed that she was able in the interview to talk about the family that she so dreaded. The following extract gives a flavour of the interview:

CN: Is this the family that you are in court with?

K: Yes, and that is ... you know you can always cut the atmosphere, with the elephant in the room that we're all not talking about and as I said I qualified a long time ago but dread them absolutely dread them every month having to go. It's um

CN: Can you talk about that because obviously that's your experience of doing home visits really? Sometimes it's useful to focus on a family and think about that.

K: Well maybe I can think about them with you but also you know the mum and the young baby as well because we did that ...

CN: That first home visit?

K: Yes. Yes. If I start with her because she can be quite interesting because she's another one that sometimes I get there and her energy levels bring my energy levels right down and it's a sort of ... you can almost feel the sort of ...

CN: And you're doing a kind of sucking motion with your mouth ... on the tape.

K: Yes well it is, she sort of sucks the life out of you and I (laughs) have to go and just getting her to sort of … it has been a struggle. I've worked with her now … for eighteen months, just over eighteen months and … there have been visits when I have been talking about really **serious** concerns around relationships with her partner and issues around the child protection plan and I'm there with sort of all the gravitas of it and saying how serious it is and then you get this flat (and I have to do the voice because it's the voice − I do it in the office laughs) sort of, oh yeah everything yeah everything and that's the response you get to anything even the most **serious** matter and I just think am I getting through to you? How am I communicating with you? But I go away thinking … I get in the car and I go …oh …

CN: And you're bodily showing me that you sag.

K: Yes, [raises voice] I do sag and I just think oh goodness me you know and I sort of go ooh … do that with my head sort of shaking my head and I just think did I get through to her at all and as I say really difficult things or it can be really positive things I'm going with and I still can get the same response. Um, it's getting slightly easier sometimes you get flashes of emotion and um response and I think maybe its the home visits that I enjoy where you get something back even if it's it's anger or discussion or something in return that you you can feed off and sort of communicate that, but you know I feel like that. If I feel like that what does her poor little son feel like and you just think poor old him, but he's such … she must be doing something really good, and she is doing something really good because his language is great and he's playing. She's going now to different groups and everything with him and her relationships she's put to one side and I think oh I must have done something in those visits when I've been you know talking to myself sometimes I used to think you know −

CN: That's what it felt like.

K: It did very much feel like I was talking to myself over and over and saying the **same** thing. That's quite disheartening going **every** visit, sometimes two, three times a week when it's really serious and saying the **same** thing over and over again but [hits table/chair] reflecting back I think well actually all that hard work you put in with her Kate has paid off because some of it must have soaked in because she's changed slowly by slowly maybe at her own pace but she has actually made progress really but … and I like her, I do like her, I've got a lot of empathy and sympathy for her. You know you know you I feel quite sorry for her because with her experiences and her child and I think she wants to be nurtured by me as well and sort of give her the positives and nurture and that's been a resistance in me because I'm **not** her mum and um don't want to be put into the mum role − having to be a bit more mum and sort of cajoling her along and sort of but it's a sort of carrot and stick with her all the time. So um −

CN: So that one sticks in your mind?

K: It does yes. She's been quite a … [chuckles] we've been on a journey together but it's doing alright but she has been just …

CN: You shake your head now.

K: It's just that voice and I, it sounds awful for me to say but its just ... you know my colleague who used to go and visit her as well and we both of us (**it's** the voice) we used share her we used to jointly work on it and it's just that sort of voice and you just I don't know if it's ... it's just ... very oh and all monotone and all everything, everything you say and I just think that is who she is you know but it isn't and I think she's starting to come out of her shell but that's ... and then my other ... [sighs]

CN: But where do you go with that when you ... you say you go in the car and ...

K: Well I go in the car and just like mutter away to myself and I talk about it all the way back and then I get back to the office and sometimes I do I like oh. [weary sigh] am I just banging my head against a brick wall and she just sits there and I have **to** say the same thing over and over and I have a bit of a rant as I do in the corner and they all roll their eyes at me and say oh right there's Kate again but and I just think oh do I have to go out again and you'll do fine and they say they give you a bit of encouragement and think about it.

CN: Did you look forward to going to see her at the time?

K: Did I look forward to it...?

CN: How does that feel when you know you've got a visit coming up?

K: ... Ah ... it ... I wouldn't say I look forward to going to see her. ... Sometimes I think what am I going to talk to her about and then I have it planned out in my head and then when you get nothing back its like ... you know I'm trying to have a social conversation with somebody and getting **nothing** in return you sort of end up talking to yourself so the time used to be ticking, **slowly** by at times and I've been thinking right I've been here thirty five minutes can I go now? [laughs]

CN: So you're kind of looking at your watch.

K: I am looking at my [laughs] watch thinking can I escape from this room and go and I used to think every time I'm finishing phew a little bit sagged – it's done but I don't have to go for maybe two weeks but other times I've gone when issues have been ... thinking right I'm going to get in there you know I'm going to get her to, really quite ... maybe that's our relationship where we've got past the platitudes.

CN: What happened when you went in like that then thinking right I'm going ... this ...?

K: I'd get a bit more from her not quite as monotone, still a bit monotone and she'd say the same things over and over again but a little more fight and she'd fight back so we'd have more of a discussion and conversation. Um cos I think it those are the times I enjoyed more because we were talking about what we needed to talk about and she was saying ... I don't mind her fighting with me, or not fighting but being more vocal in what she thinks because I'm I'm then she's telling me probably more the truth rather than what she thinks I want to hear so we can talk about it. We can talk in relation to her child and it's about supporting what we can and um empowering her to think about things – yes she wants to be in a relationship that's fine but these are the things that you need to think about within that relationship that's all I was asking her to do really and sort of the impact on her and her son So those were much easier, they were hard work I'd stay there a lot longer than the other visits but there were I felt I'd accomplished more than those ones were it was literally, yes he's been to do this and no he hasn't done that and oh I'm so tired [sighs] I want a break, I want a break, I want a break. A break from what, you know this is motherhood? So but it makes a difference. It makes a difference. Whereas the other family I absolutely dread.

CN: You've put your hand to your head like you've whacked yourself.

K: I just … I don't know I, I I think they got to me on many levels not just having to go and visit them because it was it was literally … you know they'd time me when I arrived and they'd time when I left and it all felt very orchestrated, the visit, they'd make sure it was all set up in the kitchen so actually spending some time with the child would mean me having to literally drag him out.

CN: How old is the child?

K: He's um 10. 10. Um, I started visiting him, he'd just turned nine. I spent seven months trying to get into the home they wouldn't allow me to visit. Um, started care proceedings which enabled us to have the visits. So everything was done [sighs] … I suppose we came on a difficult basis they didn't agree with us being involved at all, didn't agree with court, didn't agree with our concerns or the risk assessment. So we had that sort of battle right from the start but the visits were … the child knew nothing about why I was visiting, still doesn't know anything about why I'm visiting. So he thought that I'd just come to do this this project on keeping safe, which was mother's explanation. I'd you know I'd talked to him a little bit about what a social worker does. So throughout as I said it's like the elephant in the room, that me the dad and the mum knew and the child obviously didn't. **That** was really hard I used to absolutely dread going um and they were very nice, they were very polite – make me a cup of tea, nice home … let's talk about, social conversations about you know 'Bake Off' and cooking and the rest of it but let's not talk about what we're supposed to be talking about. You know. Now it's the politeness … that that really was going into polite society and, and being ever so, felt like ever so middle class so conversation but it was **absolutely exhausting** and I absolutely dreaded going. I used to have everybody psych me up to go and supporting me to go because it was just … just –

And:

K: … and that is … you know you can always cut the atmosphere, with the elephant in the that we're all not talking about and as I said I qualified a long time ago but dread them absolutely dread them every month having to go. It's um

CN: Well, when you're there – what does it feel like?

K: It feels awful, it feels quite lonely and it feels [sighs] … as I said I feel the tension and I feel it's quite stressful.

CN: How do you feel it because you're sort of pointing to your chest … does it affect you physically?

K: Yes because I think I used to get real pains across my back like stabbing pains um and I think I've never … **every** single sentence I'd be thinking about before I even spoke, even talking about banal things like 'Bake Off' what do I respond? I'm **really very** careful about **every** single thing I say.

Summary and comments

In Mandy's interview, the use of repetition i.e. 'cot death' times three, the hesitations, dysfluency and the affect of laughs and sighs, all serve to indicate the level of anxious arousal for her in the original encounter and how this was re-experienced within the interview itself.

Mandy was quite clear that what she encountered on this visit was not at all what she had been expecting. In the interview Mandy appeared to be particularly perplexed as to why she had not just asked the mother to turn the heating on. She seemed preoccupied with this and rationalised why she had behaved in this way. She spoke of her concerns about gaining access to this young woman and her child, as there had been information to suggest that this was an issue, as well as how being direct and forceful on a first meeting might adversely impact on the subsequent engagement and working relationship. Mandy continued to seem troubled by this, and although intellectually she could present reasons to herself as to why she had not said this, these did not appear to satisfy her. Mandy talked of how she had asked colleagues in the office on her return what they would have done.

From her account of her actions immediately following the home visit, it was clear that Mandy had sought support and containment from colleagues in the team and the team manager. Following this opportunity for 'offloading' and discussion with the team manager, Mandy then stated the actions she had taken i.e. texting the young woman and telling her to take the baby to see the GP that afternoon and to inform her (Mandy) of the outcome of the appointment, as well as a telephone conversation with the health visitor. Mandy was able to articulate that after all of the above that her anxiety which had been acute 'eased somewhat' and she was able to be thinking about planning the intervention with the family over the next few weeks.

What was apparent to me was that Mandy had needed and used her colleagues and the team manager to be able to manage the impact of the encounter with this woman and baby and that she had had to communicate and get rid of and/or 'offload' the experience in order to begin to be able to process, digest and think about what had occurred. This reduced her arousal levels and in turn allowed her to be able to think, take and plan appropriate action with the aim of safeguarding the wellbeing of a very young and vulnerable child.

The sense of Mandy carrying a burden, that is, an unpleasant experience of anxiety or concern away with her from her contact with this young mother and her baby was very powerful. As was her response in her desire to rid herself of these feelings. I contrasted this with my experience of the young woman who had presented as flat and depressed, with little energy or vitality and no expressed anxiety or concern. It seemed to me that the social worker had been invaded by and was carrying the anxiety that the young woman was not able to express.

Kate also expressed her views and feelings through physical gestures, actions and behaviours. These 'expressed somatic symptoms' occurred when she was talking about clients that appeared to have had a particularly troubling and disturbing impact on her. In turn this gave me the impression that as well as the behaviour being a form of communication it also indicated the primitive nature of the original encounter or experience, in that it was *felt, experienced and held in the body* and that to some extent it could only be re-communicated or expressed through physical and non-verbal means.

The theme of Kate feeling personally and professionally threatened in regard to the sessions with the second 'Bake Off' family was strongly transmitted. With this family my impression was that Kate experienced these encounters as traumatic and immediately threatening, so that this presented as a primary trauma.

This contrasted with Kate's description and discussion of her work with the young single mother and little boy, which had a 'deadening' impact on her. Although Kate seemed to feel drained, exhausted and frustrated by this young woman, she did not appear to feel threatened as she did with the other family. My sense therefore, was that this could be an example of the practitioner experiencing a secondary trauma, the experience of the original trauma from the client being unconsciously communicated to the practitioner.

Kate was confident enough in her skills and abilities to be able to seek and receive advice and support from her colleagues in the team and this appeared, as with Mandy, to be a very important source of emotional containment and support for her.

What the social workers were communicating

The social workers seemed to be telling me – and *showing* me – how direct contact with some service users had a profound, persistent and long lasting impact on them. That somehow certain clients had gotten under their skin so that the practitioners appeared preoccupied and inhabited by them.

The interviews were transcribed in detail and include noting differences in an interviewee's tone, volume, emphasis and non-verbal communication, hesitation, dysfluencies, etc. When noted in each of the interviews, it became very clear how significant and pervasive this 'non-verbal' communication was in their discourse.

Crittenden and Landini (2011) suggest that non-verbal or somatic behaviours – which they termed 'Expressed Somatic Symptoms' or ESS – can indicate which subjects or issues raise most anxiety for the speaker, and that 'Expressed Somatic Symptoms can be thought of as maximizing expressivity at the expense of specificity. That is the speaker "lives" the representation and imposes it strongly on the listener, but neither is clear about what it means …' (p. 273). I would add that they are not able to articulate these feelings.

The social workers did not seem particularly pleased that certain families or individuals inhabited their thoughts or preoccupied and worried them. This appeared to be a process that the workers had little or no control over and the interviews presented a safe space that allowed these issues to come to the surface and be expressed.

The ESS suggested to me that for the practitioners these troubling encounters had not been able to be fully processed so that they could not be expressed in spoken language. These experiences for the social workers were uncomfortable, unsettling and disturbing and could remain so even after periods of weeks, months or sometimes longer.

The workers appeared anxious and apprehensive about direct contact with certain families, children or individuals and they appeared keen to communicate these experiences to me as a researcher in the interviews.

What psychodynamic theory or theories might explain these phenomena?

How and why did some families or individuals have this impact on social work practitioners? What was going on in these interactions and encounters that caused the social workers to appear so preoccupied and inhabited by certain individuals or families?

In the research I explored psychoanalytic theories of unconscious defences, anxiety and resistance e.g.: repression, denial, splitting, projective identification, idealisation, acting out, turning against the self/identification with the aggressor, regression, displacement and rationalisation. Here, I suggest the reader consults a very helpful paper by Trevithick (2011) to understand and make sense of psychic defence mechanisms as likely to be experienced by social workers.

The information from the interviews lead me to me focus on the psychoanalytic concept of projective identification. This is a difficult concept to understand; not least, it seems, because in the field of psychodynamic and psychoanalytic theory different writers or clinicians may have different understandings of the term.

Hinshelwood defines projective identification as follows:

> This is the more traditional view of projection in which a part of the self is attributed to an object. Thus part of the ego – a mental state, for instance, such as unwelcome anger, hatred, or other bad feeling – is seen in another person and quite disowned (denied).
>
> *(Hinshelwood, 1989: 398)*

It was the psychoanalyst Melanie Klein (1946) who first used the phrase projective identification in relation to her theoretical basis of life and death drives and the infant's desire to take control of and/or invade or plunder the object. Klein suggested that as a way to manage the often-intense negative and positive feelings of love, anger, desire, hate, etc. the infant develops mechanisms for splitting off and projection of these feelings into an object – usually the primary care giver. This process is primitive and unconscious and is a way of dealing with emotional or physical pain or anxiety. (At this stage in their development the infant is unable to distinguish between mental pain or anxiety and uncomfortable physiological sensations – these are undifferentiated.)

Wilfred Bion (1959, 1962a, 1963, 1965, 1970), following from Klein, suggested that projective identification could also be conceived as a primitive method of communication. Bion's hypothesis was that if the object (caregiver) is able and willing to take in, receive and tolerate the projected aspects from the infant, especially any overwhelming or intolerable emotions or feelings, such as hate, aggression, anxiety, and yet maintain mental balance, then this process, if repeated consistently, allows for the emotional and cognitive development of the infant or child, including the capacity for thought. For example, when a baby cries an attuned caregiver will be able to differentiate between the cries – and certain utterances will elicit an immediate and urgent response, such as the pain cry, which is sudden and shrill. This is an example of non-verbal and primitive communication in regard to the mental state of one individual to another. I think we can probably all recall how we can be affected by the emotional state of another person and how this is automatic and out of our control. Projective identification is more than this though – it is the projection of certain emotional states into another so that the projector can deny or dissociate feeling or experiencing these troubling feelings. For the recipient this experience is usually profoundly unsettling and disturbing. Trevithick states that:

> Projective Identification describes how a person's feelings of say anger or disappointment, are located *in the practitioner* who finds him or herself unwittingly and uncharacteristically feeling confusing or unsettling emotions for no discernible reason – a situation I describe as being *mobilised* by another person to act on his/her behalf.
>
> (Trevithick, 2011: 404)

Projective identification and projection (falsely attributed thoughts, feelings, attributes, etc. projected on to someone or something else) are unconscious processes that, especially for projective identification, are primarily defensive in nature; that is, they defend the individual against unbearable psychic pain, anxiety or conflict. In the interviews an example could be when Mandy appears to be full of anxiety for the four-month-old baby, when the baby's mother presents as flat and depressed.

How does this work? By what mechanism can the internal state of one person be transferred or impact another?

Schore, writing in 2002, referenced psychoanalytic theory and research in neuroscience to propose how this phenomena works and suggests:

A fundamental principle of my work is that no theory of emotional development can be restricted to only a description of psychological processes; it must
also be consonant with what we now know about the biological structure of
the brain.

(Schore and Sieff, 2015: 112)

And:

An integrative model is proposed which suggests that projective identification
is an early appearing yet enduring intra-psychic mechanism that mediates the
unconscious transmission of psychobiological states between the right brains of
both members of an affect communicating dyad.

(Schore, 2002: 1)

Schore, referring to Klein (1946), proposes that projective identification emerges
very early in life as a primitive form of communication between the infant and
caregiver, which involves communication between the unconscious of both and
that: 'Primitive mental states ... are more precisely characterized as *psychobiological
states*' (Schore, 2002: 4).

Schore argues that at this stage of development, primitive mental states are
inseparable from the physical state and are experienced as such, so that distress for
the infant is experienced as pain and communicated through the body. He proposes that it is in this way – understanding this from a 'psychobiological' perspective – that 'affective' states are transmitted between infant and caregiver and states
that: 'This highly efficient system of somatically driven, fast acting emotional
communication is essentially nonverbal' (Schore, 2002: 3).

Schore cites neuro-scientific research which has demonstrated that different areas
of the brain are involved in management of different functions, i.e. the right side of
the brain is involved with recognising and responding to affect or emotional states
or communications – embodied and non-verbal cues such as facial expression,
gesture, posture, tone and volume of voice, etc. The left side of the brain is
dedicated to the symbolic cognitive, i.e. use and interpretation of language.

Schore proposes that in early development, prior to the infant being able to use
symbolic expression or interpretation (language), that affect and emotional and
feeling states are communicated through right brain to right brain functioning and
that these exchanges are very fast and below the 'radar' of conscious awareness.
Schore goes on to describe projective identification as:

an early organizing unconscious coping strategy for regulating right-brain to
right-brain communications especially that of intense affective states. Since
affects are psychobiological phenomena and the self is bodily based, the coping
strategy of projective identification represents non conscious verbal linguistic
behaviours but unconscious nonverbal *mind-body communications*.

(Schore, 2002: 8)

As the infant communicates affective states through non-verbal means, it requires a reliably receptive and responsive care giver, who can receive, accept and contain these communications and respond in a manner that allows for the infant to experience a lessening or alleviating of the felt pain and discomfort. This could be through, touch, sound, holding, feeding, etc.

However, Schore suggests that where the infant experiences adverse care or abuse, in that the communication of affective states is not responded to or receives a negative response, that the infant will, if this situation continues or if the affective state becomes so intense that it is overwhelming, switch to a dissociative state: that is, close down emotionally and physically with the aim of regulation and return to some sort of homeostatic balance. He suggests that this pattern of unconscious functioning can then become established and persist as the infant develops.

Thus, projective identification can be understood as a primitive mechanism for communicating and transmitting information on affective states between two people, usually someone that the infant is in a close, intimate (physical and psychological) relationship with. This is a phenomenon that occurs when one is in close physical proximity with another – or where it is possible to see, hear, feel, even smell, non-verbal cues and actions.

Schore argues that this phenomena is repeated in the therapeutic encounter, with the therapist in the role of the mother or care giver to the 'infant' and that this will be disturbing for the therapist as the transmission (through projective identification) will be unconsciously picked up by the right brain and experienced in the body of the therapist (due to the right brain's connection to the limbic system).

In addition, he states, that the moment of projective identification is the shift, the switch, from an intensely dysregulated state to a disassociative one, with the effect that the therapist experiences a sense of the dysregulation, but the patient is 'cut off' from this state and may give no sign of it – as seen, I suggest, in Mandy's encounter with the young mother and baby.

Schore also links the phenomena of projective identification as encountered in psychotherapy sessions with experiences of early trauma (especially in relation to attachment figures or relationships), which occurred prior to the development of language and such that the impressions, memory, recollection in relation to the original emotional state is not part of a narrative able to be described in language, but is triggered in the relationship and interaction with the therapist and 'relived' in the sessions (Schore, 2012: 169). Schore is clear that this is not just a psychic communication between two minds – of the patient and the therapist – but between *two bodies* (Schore, 2012: 179). The communications are projected, received, experienced in the bodies of the patient and the analyst and that this is primarily unconscious and automatic as processed by the right brain and limbic system.

Schore's work, as referenced above, pertains to the analytic endeavour and implications for clinical practice. However, the research and theory as outlined above are equally applicable when considering the data that emerged in my research project.

Link to trauma

Schore makes a link between the phenomena of projective identification and early trauma for the patient and I also considered the relevance of trauma in the research. Both primary and secondary trauma (Garland, 1998; Pearlman, 1995) were examined as theories that might assist in making sense of encounters between the practitioners and their clients. It seemed that direct encounters with some clients could be experienced as traumatic for the social workers. This may be linked to experiences of early trauma for the client, but also that the encounters themselves, dealing with hostility and aggression, were a primary trauma for practitioners. It appeared from the data as though the social workers were compelled at some level to replay and rehearse their troubled and troubling encounters with clients, including in the interviews.

Some of the symptoms of stress the social workers talked about in their interviews suggested not that they were experiencing a secondary trauma, but actually their experience was of a primary traumatic experience, as their minds and psychic structure and integrity were threatened and assaulted *in the sessions*. The clients appeared to be resistant to social work intervention and defended against what this represented for them.

Defended subjects

In the research I suggested that it was the encounters with individuals or families with the most intense psychic defences that were most difficult for practitioners. Unlike patients in therapy, who have given their consent to therapeutic intervention, clients of statutory children's services are most often involuntary recipients of the service. This in my view suggests that the psychic defences may be even more prevalent and intense than for recipients of therapy, including and perhaps especially the use of projective identification.

Social workers must often struggle to overcome the defences in their direct work with children and families. They have to gain access and then seek to engage with and develop positive working relationships with individuals and families. Greater awareness of the impact that psychic defences have on undertaking the social work task could have significant implications for practice in considering how interventions might be made more effective. From this research it appeared that the psychic defences and the levels of anxiety within a family were directly correlated with the anxiety levels and emotional state of the social worker.

It appeared that the phenomena as recounted by the practitioners in this project had their origins with specific clients. This was evidenced by the fact that, when working with certain families, the practitioners experienced the encounters quite differently, and there was a marked contrast in how they experienced working with the families that they appeared to be preoccupied and inhabited by in the interviews.

These troublesome or 'toxic' families appeared to be exceptional, but were routinely experienced in the team and the organisation (and external agencies such as health and legal services) as difficult and challenging and acknowledged as such. An example of this would be the second family Kate talked about in her interview.

What happens to the child?

What was noticeable in the social worker's discourse in the interviews was that when preoccupied and 'inhabited' by certain clients, how the child, the subject of the intervention, appeared to slip from view, and the struggle by the social worker to maintain their focus on the child or children when caught up in the defensive behaviours and projections of the adult or adults involved. As Syed states: 'Attention … is a scarce resource: if you focus on one thing you will lose awareness of other things.' (Syed, 2015: 29). The child may be the subject of the intervention and his/her interests must be the paramount consideration at all times (HM Government, 2015). However, there is an immediate difficulty that seemed evident in the discourse of the practitioners; that is, whilst the child or children are the subjects of the intervention and their needs must be kept as 'paramount', it is the *adults, the parents or caregivers* that are expected to change (their behaviours/attitudes/actions) for the benefit of the child. And it is with the adults that the social work practitioner has to engage or develop some kind of relationship, most times even before they can meet with the child or children.

The relevance for social work practitioners as evidenced from the data that emerged in this research project is that the same or similar process occurs in direct encounters with certain clients as is experienced in psychoanalytic encounters, so that intense defensive reactions (usually from adult parents or care givers) can have an impact on the ability of the social worker to undertake the tasks assigned to them. This includes being able to maintain the focus on the child or children. Harry Ferguson wrote an article for the *Guardian* in 2013 on why social workers (SWs) become 'helpless' and children become 'invisible'. Ferguson referred to his research and related how:

> On one home visit the SW, faced by an angry mother denying child neglect, completely ignored the two children that were right in front of her. Another SW failed to challenge a belligerent father about the neglect she had found, and did not see the children … on their own. Afterwards she spoke vividly about how she felt the neglected house – especially the smell – overcame her.
>
> *(Ferguson, 2013)*

It seems that the negative impact of these projections on the practitioner may not only effect how the social worker assesses or interacts with the child or children in that particular family, but may have a knock-on effect on their capacity to work with other children and families. That is, when the impact of projections and encounters with certain clients is so profound and intense, the practitioner's functioning, cognitive and physiological, is affected so that their capacity to focus on, attend to and carry out other tasks, including work with *other families and children*, could be adversely impacted. If one considers that practitioners will often visit more than one family or child in a day, it is not difficult to appreciate how a disturbing encounter with a client such as described in the social work interviews would continue beyond the period of the actual session and impact on subsequent visits or sessions and likely impair assessments, judgement and decision making.

It appeared that without adequate time and conditions for recovery and processing this could then impact on the practitioner's capacity to complete other tasks, including assessing situations and risk for other children and families over a longer term.

The role of the organisation

The role of the organisation, both practically in allowing and encouraging practitioners to talk openly about their experiences, without fear of censure or compromising their career or position, as well as in terms of the 'organisation-in-the-mind' (Armstrong, 1991) that workers carry with them as internalised ideals and ethos, appears from this research to be of critical importance in managing and dealing with the emotional impact of direct work.

Evidence from the practitioners interviewed suggested that they had an acute need to use the organisation to assist them with managing and processing the impact of the work, especially direct work with intense and troubling projections from clients. It is to the organisation, their colleagues, the team and the manager to which the practitioners appeared *to turn to first* to assist them to manage and process these difficult and disturbing encounters. If the response they receive is experienced as positive and containing, then the practitioners appeared more enabled to proceed and manage and process the emotional impact of the work, including being able to think, reflect and take action where appropriate. *This suggests that the role of the organisation is of critical importance in enabling the practitioner to retain (or regain) the focus on the child.*

Therefore I suggest that the organisation needs to be structured in such a way that addresses this and in a manner that encourages and facilitates thinking and creativity through providing safe and containing environments where these troubling and disturbing aspects of the work can be acknowledged and processed.

Implications for practice

This research indicated that one immediate way to assist practitioners would be for research to confirm their own experiences; that the impact of direct work can be profoundly disturbing and generally the origin of this disturbance is related to the psychic defences of the client, not a personal failing or weakness in individual workers. These phenomena, if confirmed, should be recognised and acknowledged as a real and frequent occurrence in practice. I propose that these phenomena should be thought of as being akin to 'turbulence' in the aviation industry: that is, a natural and regularly occurring phenomena which requires consistent responses from trained and experienced personnel in order to minimise risk of injury (International Air Transport Association, 2015). The analogy for me is particularly appropriate, as although turbulence is common and to a certain degree can be predicted, the individual incidents will not be exactly the same and some incidents will be much more severe than others, and some perhaps will occur without any warning.

If practitioners are able to feel that they have permission to talk more openly about their personal experiences in working with children and their families, without fear of censure or blame then this may minimise any sense of shame. This, in turn, may have a beneficial effect on the social worker's capacity for creativity when undertaking the primary task.

If the phenomena of projective identification and primary and secondary trauma can be better understood in the social work context, then I would hope that the negative impact of some of these disturbing encounters could be 'de-toxified' to some extent. This would assist the practitioners, but could also improve the service to the children and families, as the clients or service users may feel more contained and supported by social workers if these phenomena could be considered as communications in regard to anxiety and early trauma and loss. This could, in my view, go a long way in counteracting the negative impact of direct work with some very difficult and challenging clients.

For instance, if these phenomena could be openly recognised and acknowledged, then strategies could be thought about and then employed to manage them. For example, in working with a particular family, where the mother has a personality disorder, and whose impact on the children's social workers has been profound due to the level and intensity of the negative projections to them, it was suggested that the case work could be organised so that a senior worker takes on the role of the direct contact with the mother, freeing up the social workers to focus on the issues for the individual children, in order that their needs and wishes do not get lost or subsumed in their mother's intense and negative projections and communications with the agency.

Arrangements such as these would require agreement from middle and senior management in terms of deployment of resources as well as close coordination between the professional team, so it would need to be sanctioned and supported by all levels of the organisation. Joint working in certain cases may also be another strategy to work with particular families where this phenomena has been identified. This too would require similar agreement and support within the organisation, but it has been my experience that practitioners value highly the experience of joint working with a colleague. This would also afford the possibility of increasing the skills and resources within social work teams, developing team support and cohesion as well as potential way of being able to address the more problematic defensive encounters with children and families.

Work discussion groups

Work discussion groups could provide a suitable space for reflection on the task and emotional impact of the work. Sometimes also named Reflective Practice

Groups, there are a number of different models including 'Critical Reflection' (Fook and Gardner 2007, 2013); 'Relationship-Based' (Ruch 2007a, 2007b, 2009); and 'Work Discussion' (Jackson, 2005; Warman and Jackson, 2007; Jackson 2008, Rustin and Bradley, 2008).

Fook and Gardner (2007) have highlighted that there has been limited evaluation of the effectiveness of Reflective Practice Groups, regardless of what model has been used. Such research would be useful to determine value to the participants (as well as to the organisation and services users) and identify advantages or disadvantages of any of the different models. Warman and Jackson (2007) have suggested that work discussion groups may have a value for social work practitioners, but this is an area in which further research is required to determine which approaches may be most effective.

Social work training

The emotional impact of direct encounters could and should be addressed as a core part of any social work training programme. Social work educators should be open and upfront with students about the situations they are likely to encounter and how this can impact on them emotionally and physically. The theory behind these experiences should be covered through work discussion, role play etc. so that practitioners can prepare for direct work and be familiar with strategies of how to manage and deal with the dynamics in difficult encounters whilst maintaining the focus on the child.

Conclusion

Direct work with families and children can have a powerful and long-lasting negative impact on practitioners, that affects their capacity to think and respond as well as invoking physiological changes akin to a stress response. Psychoanalytic theory and research in neuroscience as combined by Schore (2002, 2012; Schore and Sieff, 2015) presents an explanation of the cognitive and physiological processes involved.

These encounters, I argue, are routine in the field of social work and practitioners require ongoing support to manage and process these experiences to minimise negative impact. This should include acknowledgement and awareness within the organisation to assist the social workers to process their experiences as well as readily available reflective supervision and ongoing training and group work with colleagues.

Editors' afterword

In this piece of research Charlotte Noyes conducted in-depth interviews of social workers who had been carrying out home visits in difficult childcare cases. She demonstrates vividly the emotional and physical impact this work has on the practitioners who urgently needed support from their colleagues or managers when they returned to the office.

This response indicates the power of the clients' projections into the worker, and Noyes points out that, when inhabited this way by the parent, it is difficult to focus on the child. Noyes suggests that social work courses should prepare students better for the reality of the work. We would add that social work courses need to teach theory which will enable the students to process their experiences in the real world.

One social worker talks about visiting a mother with a young child: 'I'm trying to have a social conversation with somebody and getting nothing in return. You sort of end up talking to yourself, so the time used to be ticking, slowly.' Here the worker is talking about her countertransference. The client is projecting into her the awfulness of being alone with a small child.

Awareness of this would have given the worker the opportunity to process this material in the way that Bion describes in his concept of containment. If the worker does not have the capacity or knowledge to do this, the client's projections can enter the worker's body as physical manifestations. We are convinced that high sickness rates in social work are at least partly due to the unprocessed experiences with clients.

Bibliography

Armstrong, D. (1991) *The Institution in the Mind: Reflections on the Relation of Psychoanalysis to Work with Institutions*. London: The Grubb Institute.

Armstrong, D. (2003) *Organisation in the Mind: Psychoanalysis, Group Relations, and Organisational Consultancy*. London, New York: Karnac.

Bion, W.R. (1959) *Experiences in Groups*. New York: Basic Books.

Bion, W.R. (1962a) A theory of thinking. In *Second Thoughts*. London: Karnac, pp. 110–119.

Bion, W.R. (1962b) *Learning from Experience*. London: Heinemann.

Bion, W.R. (1963) *Elements of Psychoanalysis*. London: Heinemann.

Bion, W.R. (1965) *Transformations*. London: Heinemann.

Bion, W.R. (1967) *Second Thoughts*. London: Maresfield.

Bion, W.R. (1970) *Attention and Interpretation*. London: Tavistock.

Bower, M. (ed.) (2005) *Psychoanalytic Theory for Social Work Practice: Thinking Under Fire*. London, New York: Routledge.

Crittenden, P.M. and Landini, A. (2011) *Assessing Adult Attachment*. New York, London: Norton.

Department for Education (2015) *Characteristics of Children in Need: 2014 to 2015*. London: UK Government.

Ferguson, H. (2003) Welfare, social exclusion and reflexivity: the case of child and woman protection. *Journal of Social Policy* 32(2), 199–216.

Ferguson, H. (2004) *Protecting Children in Time: Child Abuse, Child Protection and the Consequences of Modernity*. Basingstoke: Palgrave.

Ferguson, H. (2005) Working with violence, the emotions and the psycho-social dynamics of child protection: reflections on the Victoria Climbie case. *Social Work Education* 24(7), 781–795.

Ferguson, H. (2007) Abused and looked-after children as 'moral dirt': child abuse and institutional care in historical perspective. *Journal of Social Policy* 36(1), 123–139.

Ferguson, H. (2008) Liquid social work: welfare interventions as mobile practices. *British Journal of Social Work* 38, 561–579.

Ferguson, H. (2009) Performing child protection: home visiting, movement and the struggle to reach the abused child. *Child and Family Social Work* 14, 471–480.

Ferguson, H. (2010) Therapeutic journeys: the car as a vehicle for working with children and families and theorizing practice. *Journal of Social Work Practice* 24(2), 121–138.

Ferguson, H. (2011a) *Child Protection Practice*. Basingstoke: Palgrave.

Ferguson, H. (2011b) The mobilities of welfare: the case of social work. In Buscher, M., Urry, J. and Witchger, J. (eds) *Mobile Methods*. London: Routledge.

Ferguson, H. (2013) Daniel Pelka: why social workers become 'helpless'. *The Guardian*, 24 September.

Ferguson, H. (2014) What social workers do in performing child protection work: evidence from research into face-to-face practice. *Child and Family Social Work* 21(3), 283–294.

Fook, J. and Gardner, F. (2007) *Practising Critical Reflection: A Resource Handbook*. Maidenhead: McGraw Hill Education and Open University Press.

Fook, J. and Gardner, F. (eds) (2013) *Critical Reflection in Context: Applications in Health and Social Care*. London, New York: Routledge.

Garland, C. (ed.) (1998) *Understanding Trauma: A Psychoanalytical Approach*. London: Tavistock Series, Duckworth.

Hinshelwood, R.D. (1989) *A Dictionary of Kleinian Thought*. London: Free Association Books.

HM Government (2015) *Working Together to Safeguard Children: A Guide to Inter-Agency Working to Safeguard and Promote the Welfare of Children*. London: UK Government.

Hoggett, P. (2000) *Emotional Life and the Politics of Welfare*. London: Macmillan.

International Air Transport Association (2015) *Guidance on Turbulence Management*. Second Edition. Available from: www.iata.org [accessed 6 February 2016].

Jackson, E. (2005) Developing observation skills in school settings: the importance and impact of 'work discussion' groups for staff. *International Journal of Infant Observation* 8(1), 5–17.

Jackson, E. (2008) The development of work discussion groups in educational settings. *Journal of Child Psychotherapy* 34(1), 62–82.

Jones, R. (2014a) *The Story of Baby P: Setting the Record Straight*. Bristol, Chicago: Policy Press.

Jones, R. (2014b) Child protection: 40 years of learning but where next? In Blyth, M. (ed.) *Moving on from Munro: Improving Children's Services*. Bristol, Chicago: Policy Press.

Klein, M. (1946) Notes on some schizoid mechanisms. In Mitchell, J. (ed.) *The Selected Melanie Klein*. London: Penguin.

Mattinson, J. (1975) *The Reflection Process in Casework Supervision*. London: TIMS.

Mattinson, J. and Sinclair, I. (1979) *Mate and Stalemate*. London, Guilford, Worcester: IMS.

Munro, E. (2005) A systems approach to investigating child abuse deaths. *British Journal of Social Work* 35, 531–546.

Munro, E. (2011a) *Second Interim Report*. London: UK Government.

Munro, E. (2011b) *The Munro Review of Child Protection. Final Report: A Child-Centred System*. London: UK Government.

Parton, N. (1985) *The Politics of Child Abuse*. Basingstoke: Macmillan.

Parton, N. (1991) *Governing the Family: Child Care, Child Protection and the State*. Basingstoke: Macmillan.

Parton, N. (1996a) Child protection, family support and social work: a critical appraisal of the Department of Health research studies in child protection. *Child and Family Social Work* 1, 3–11.

Parton, N. (ed.) (1996b) *Social Theory, Social Change and Social Work: The State of Welfare*. London, New York: Routledge.

Parton, N. (2008) Changes in the form of knowledge in social work: from the 'social' to the 'informational'. *British Journal of Social Work* 38(2), 253–269.

Parton, N. (2012) The Munro review of child protection: an appraisal. *Children and Society* 26, 150–162.

Parton, N. (2014) *The Politics of Child Protection: Contemporary Developments and Future Directions*. London: Palgrave Macmillan.

Parton, N., Thorpe, D. and Wattam, C. (1997) *Child Protection, Risk and the Moral Order*. Basingstoke: Macmillan.

Pearlman, L.A. (1995) Notes from the field: Laurie Anne Pearlman what is vicarious Traumatization? In Hudnall Stamm, B. (ed.) *Secondary Traumatic Stress: Self-Care Issues for Clinicians, Researchers and Educators*. Baltimore: Sidran Press, pp. xlvii–lii.

Preston-Shoot, M. and Agass, D. (1990) *Making Sense of Social Work: Psychodynamics, Systems and Practice*. London: Macmillan.

Ruch, G. (2007a) Reflective practice in contemporary child-care social work: The role of containment. *British Journal of Social Work* 37, 659–680.

Ruch, G. (2007b) 'Thoughtful' practice: child-care social work and the role of case discussion. *Child and Family Social Work* 12, 370–379.

Ruch, G. (2009) Identifying 'the critical' in a relationship based model of reflection. *European Journal of Social Work* 12(3), 349–362.

Ruch, G., Turney, D. and Ward, A. (eds.) (2010) *Relationship-Based Social Work: Getting to the Heart of Practice*. London, Philadelphia: Jessica Kingsley.

Rustin, M. and Bradley, J. (eds) (2008) *Work Discussion: Learning from Reflective Practice in Work with Children and Families*. London: Karnac.

Schore, A.N. (2000) Attachment and the regulation of the right brain. *Attachment and Human Development* 2(1), 23–47.

Schore, A.N. (2002) Clinical implications of a psychoneurobiological model of projective identification. In Alhanati, S. (ed.) *Primitive Mental States Volume II: Psychobiological and Psychoanalytic Perspectives on Early Trauma and Personality Development*. New York, London: Karnac, pp. 1–66.

Schore, A.N. (2012) *The Science of the Art of Psychotherapy*. New York, London: W.W. Norton and Company.

Schore, A.N. and Sieff, D. (2015) On the same wave-length: how our emotional brain is shaped by human relationships. In Sieff, D. (ed.) *Understanding and Healing Emotional Trauma: Conversations with Pioneering Clinicians and Researchers*. London, New York: Routledge, pp. 111–136.

Syed, M. (2015) *Black Box Thinking: The Surprising Truth About Success (and Why Some People Never Learn from Their Mistakes)*. London: John Murray.

Trevithick, P. (2011) Understanding defences and defensiveness in social work. *Journal of Social Work Practice* 25(4), pp. 389–412.

Trevithick, P. and Wengraf, T. (2011) Special issue: defences and defensiveness. *Journal of Social Work Practice* 25(4), 383–387.

Warman, A. and Jackson, E. (2007) Recruiting and retaining children and families' social workers: the potential of work discussion groups. *Journal of Social Work Practice* 21(1), 35–48.

Warner, J. (2015) *The Emotional Politics of Social Work and Child Protection*. Bristol, New York: Policy Press.

5

REFLECTIVE SUPERVISION FOR CHILD PROTECTION PRACTICE

Researching beneath the surface

Anna Harvey and Fiona Henderson

It is increasingly recognised that attending to the emotional aspects of social work is a vital component of supervision (Munro, 2011). However, there is a danger that we can adopt a rather dichotomous view of supervision where it is regarded as either nurturing or controlling, all about feelings or all about procedure. This is a reflection of the tensions inherent in the profession between developing expertise and managing performance, which may replicate care and control splits in child protection work with families. These splits may be realistic and the requirements of managerial versus professional supervision may simply be incompatible. Opportunities for emotional attuning and reflection on cases cannot be tagged on to performance checks in a token way and we need to be clearer about the theoretical frameworks which support the models of supervision we are delivering. Likewise the content of supervision cannot be reduced to a tick-box exercise with reflection or critical analysis being compartmentalised. The Professional Capabilities Framework (PCF) informing support and assessment for newly qualified staff may lend itself to this kind of reductionism.

In this chapter, we present a case study of psychoanalytically informed reflective supervision with a social worker to illustrate how the model works in practice. We follow the supervision of 'Nadine', a newly qualified social worker, on the Assessed and Supported Year in Employment (ASYE) post-qualifying training. (In order to preserve anonymity, Nadine and the case described are amalgamated from supervision situations encountered over many years.) Nadine was supervised on a weekly basis for a year by an independent supervisor (AH) from outside her organisation. The supervision was commissioned to provide an opportunity for reflection on her cases as opposed to a more managerial, task-orientated approach. All decision-making powers were retained by her line manager while the reflective supervision provided her with a thinking space to help deepen her practice. The supervision provided a level of consistency and security for Nadine in a chaotic and ever-changing organisation (six line managers had come and gone by the end of her first year). This model offered a reliable framework to support her learning and meant that she had someone who she could depend and rely upon. By seeing her supervisor consistently in this way she was able to become more sensitive to the families she worked with and her assessments were more effective as a result of the insights she gained.

A clinical approach to supervision

Bower (2003, 2005) emphasises the importance of having a strong and applicable theory base to underpin social work practice. It must have sufficient depth to reflect the complex realities of the work and to help us make sense of the impact the work has on us. She points out that although 'emotional disturbance and the power of the unconscious internal world' have been marginalised in social work training, they are integral parts of a client's experience (Bower, 2005: 3). Bower describes how unconscious communications make themselves felt in the relationships between client and worker and these feelings can have a profound and destabilising effect on us. The emotional impact on the worker can be obvious or subtle, resulting in feelings like confusion, despair and anger. We might also find ourselves acting in ways that we do not recognise as our own, such as becoming overly harsh or indulgent towards clients (Bower, 2005: 4).

In her paper 'Broken and Twisted' Bower describes the way in which the structure and framework of a year-long, post-qualifying course provided a containing function for social workers, where their needs for dependability and consistency were met (Bower, 2003). In turn, the workers were able to become more sensitive to the needs of the children they saw. This model can be replicated in reflective supervision by providing the same kind of containment, promoted by a consistent setting and familiar person who has an available mind, which is open to the emotional experiences of the practitioner. It is helpful if the supervisor has some distance from the pressures of the organisation, and can therefore provide a different, more clinical point of view. This also helps the social worker think about the wider organisational dynamics which they may be responding to. The supervision maintains a focus on the child's experience, as this is frequently lost in the scramble to meet the needs of parents who are often deprived, vulnerable themselves and requiring a great deal of support.

Social workers often find it difficult to keep both the adult and child in mind as a connected pair, and the pressures of the child protection system can create a sense that they are somehow competing. This is reflected in some case discussions with social workers where the child is rarely mentioned or is poorly described. Very often the parents' needs can overwhelm the social worker so that they have little space left in their minds to think about the children. This can be a version of how the parents also feel and it can be helpful to disentangle these parallel processes during supervision.

Containment through supervision

Containment is a psychoanalytic concept developed by Wilfred Bion drawing on Melanie Klein's earlier work on projective processes in infancy. Containment is an interpersonal process which lies at the heart of communication and empathy. It originates in the relationship between a baby and its mother. In a healthy situation, a baby will evacuate (or project) feeling-states, like confusion and fear, into its mother who will feel them herself. The difference is that the mother will be able to use her mind to think about these states and, in so doing, transform them into more bearable experiences for her baby. With repeated 'containment' of this kind, the baby will develop a capacity to tolerate greater uncertainty and distress by themselves but importantly, this is a struggle that endures throughout life.

Projection is an unconscious process in the mind which strives to rid us of uncomfortable or unwanted feelings, such as anxiety or helplessness, often by attributing them to others. A person on the receiving end of projections begins to experience these feelings as their own, becoming 'identified' with them through a process called projective identification.

For example, during a home visit a social worker talks to a mother who is feeling ashamed because she views herself as inadequate and failing as a parent. As a defence, the mother projects her unwanted feelings into the social worker whom she now regards as useless. In turn the social worker is affected by the projections and for a while feels pretty hopeless herself. This is a common experience in social work, where the client fears judgement from outside as well as from within themselves; in response, the client turns the tables and evokes a bad feeling in the social worker, converting fears about being 'a bad parent' into finding fault with professional practice. This may affect social workers' decision-making about a case, for example not visiting again, transferring the case to another team and feeling relieved not to see the family any more.

This same struggle in the social worker may also be a response to a profound feeling of despair in the parent which is being communicated unconsciously. Supervision can help to make sense of these powerful emotions and bring awareness that the feelings belong to the parent and not the practitioner, reflecting some of their deepest worries. This might allow the social worker to visit the mother again and convey an understanding of how she may be feeling at a loss to know what to do with her child. The mother may feel relief that she has been understood and that her strong negative feelings have been survived. This is an experience of containment. The client has been helped to manage a difficult or painful belief about themselves through projective processes, leading to an understanding between worker and client and a discovery of what is going on. This process of making meaning can help to support necessary insight and change.

In a similar way, reflective supervision can provide an opportunity for containment of a practitioner's anxieties resulting from the raw experience of the work. Through close listening to the case material, the supervisor takes in the rawness and transforms it into thoughts and ideas which are reflected back to bring understanding of the client's situation. The supervisor puts themselves in the way of the workers' projections to pick up on the emotional resonances evoked by the case and to start to have ideas about what might be significant for that client. This is similar to the concept of countertransference which refers to the strong emotional responses we can have to a case. As Bion described, we project feelings that we are struggling with, not only to rid ourselves of them, but in order to communicate these feelings to others. If we can examine the impact that a family has upon us then we may be able to reach a deeper level of understanding about their hopes and fears.

This chapter explores the unconscious processes that were evoked by one particularly difficult case in order to highlight the containing function of the supervision, not only for the practitioner but also for the family as a whole. We describe how individual practitioners or whole teams can unintentionally enact parts in the drama of a case, reflecting the fragmented internal world of the client or family's situation. In so doing, professionals can develop 'symptoms' of the family's disturbance which are often signalled by:

> intensity of feeling aroused by a case; the degree of dogmatism evoked; or the pressure to take drastic or urgent measures or expressed in action through responses such as inappropriate unconcern; surprising ignorance; undue complacency; uncharacteristic insensitivity or professional inertia.
>
> (Britton, 2005: 165)

The case study illustrates how feelings of fear and guilt were stirred in a social worker during the course of her work and how these feelings were worked with in supervision.

Case study

A social worker, 'Nadine', brought a case to supervision involving a five-week-old baby 'Ayesha', who was removed from her mother's care at birth. The baby's mother was an 18-year-old woman called 'Tanya'. Tanya was in a relationship with 'Dan,' a 46-year-old man, who was not the biological father of Ayesha, but who wished to raise the child as his own. Tanya and Dan became involved in a relationship when Tanya was just a few months pregnant. However, they had known each other a long time, as Dan had been in a relationship with her mother when Tanya was 13 years old. Dan was a heroin and crack user and was alleged to have injected Tanya with heroin. Tanya had experienced extreme maternal deprivation as a child and had been severely emotionally and physically abused. She had been in and out of care whilst growing up.

Tanya's 'chaotic lifestyle' and difficulties with alcohol misuse meant that Ayesha was made subject to a child protection plan prior to birth. She was then placed in foster care on an Interim Care Order when she was born. Tanya had supervised contact with Ayesha for three hours, four days a week in the foster carer's home and on an additional day Dan attended contact with her at a local centre.

Nadine had been allocated this case just prior to the baby's birth and she had little time to formulate a pre-birth assessment. The first meeting she had with Tanya was to tell her that the baby would be removed from her care. Following the removal Nadine had to assess what the next steps were going to be; whether Ayesha could be returned home to a safe enough environment following work with the parents or whether she should be placed permanently in adoptive care. Nadine had been asked by the court to undertake a short 'viability assessment' to decide whether Ayesha and Tanya should move into a mother and baby unit together, as Tanya had made an application for a residential parenting assessment. The pressure to make final decisions about the care plan were huge as care proceedings take place within a strict 26 week timeframe.

Home visit – 'That's a knife, a big knife, a very, very big knife'

Nadine was asked to complete detailed written accounts of some of her home visits to bring to supervision. The aim was to record her observations of a visit in as much detail as possible including her spontaneous reactions, hunches and questions. These would be read out loud by Nadine to the supervision group and then read again in silence in order for us to digest the information more carefully. This careful approach slowed down our thinking, opening us up to emotional responses to the case and enabling us to pick up on possible meanings beneath the surface of the interactions between people as we were hearing about them. This way of recording the process of a meeting with a client is based on the 'work discussion group' developed at the Tavistock Clinic, and its purpose is to bring to light the unconscious meanings in the work (Rustin and Bradley, 2008).

The process recording of a home visit presented below was an account of Nadine's third and last meeting with Tanya before compiling her viability report. Tanya had missed contact with Ayesha on the morning of the home visit. Before the visit Nadine was already anxious that Dan may be threatening towards her as he had been angry with her over the telephone. He had interpreted her discussions with Tanya about going into a mother and baby unit as an attempt to split them up. Nadine decided to arrange a joint home visit with her manager. This is Nadine's process recording:

> Before the visit I had to wait for the manager for 35 minutes as he was late. He complained that someone had blocked him into the car park and he was unable to leave on time. When we went into the family home I felt scared. It was quite dark and no one was in the front room. I called hello and Dan came out of the bedroom, I thought looking red and a bit high. He said that Tanya was in the bedroom and we looked in. She was in bed looking dazed, opening and closing her mouth, as if dehydrated. She had a big bruise on her shoulder and some on her arms, which she tried to hide with her nightie. I observed a used condom on the cabinet next to the bed and there was a pungent mixture of smells from alcohol, sex and personal neglect. The manager asked if I could give him a minute to talk privately with Tanya and I went into the front room with Dan. I asked Dan if they had been drinking the night before and he said they had and Tanya had been very drunk.

He said that they had had a 'blow up' and the police had been called by a neighbour. Four policemen had turned up and had told him to leave. I asked about the bruises on Tanya's arms and he said they were grip marks as he had to stop her from self-harming. He went into the kitchen and got the kitchen knife that she had tried to cut herself with. It was over a foot long and I felt my face drain with shock, thinking that I shouldn't show him how scared I was and hope that he would put it back quickly. I had seen this knife at the previous visit on the kitchen bench but I had 'forgotten' about it. I was able to ask Dan in a half jokey manner, whether he was threatening me with the knife and this seemed to diffuse the situation, as he laughed and said of course not putting it away again.

Dan left the flat and I went through to the bedroom. The manager was advising Tanya that she should go to the GP because of a pain she had. He said Tanya was too ill to take part in my meeting. I asked Tanya if she wanted me to come back another time and she said she was fine to talk to me now, getting up and joining me and the manager on the sofa. I told Tanya that Dan had told me what happened the previous night and that she had got very drunk. When I was talking to Tanya, trying to get her version of what happened the manager yawned and interrupted the conversation. I continued with my questions and Tanya revealed that she had arranged to meet up with her ex-partner for some 'excitement'. She smiled as she told us what had happened and I thought she had enjoyed the drama of the night before. I pointed out that she had missed her contact with Ayesha because she had gone out and got drunk.

The manager told me that he had to leave and I continued talking to Tanya who was able to give me quite a detailed account of her history. I received a message from the manager later in the day saying he had found the home visit very disturbing. When I eventually met with him the next day I told him about the knife. He laughed and questioned whether the knife was really as big as I said. He was vague about the action I might take. The manager made it clear that he viewed Dan as a 'good man' who was trying to support his partner. He considered him as the more responsible of the two.

After the visit I thought about Ayesha who I had seen at her foster carers the day before. I thought about how tiny and vulnerable she was and how a five-week-old baby would fare in this kind of home. I had the awful thought that if Ayesha were to be returned she would be at risk of being killed by her parents, accidentally or not, whilst in a drunken state. Even the mere thought that the baby could be returned home now seemed a mad proposition and I felt acutely embarrassed that I had ever contemplated it. I thought about the enormity of what I was being asked to do, and wondered whether I was capable of taking the responsibility involved to make decisions about such huge matters. I felt very alone with it all, despite being part of a multi-disciplinary team and co-working the case with my manager.

Supervision discussion

Counter-transference

During supervision we discussed how the most worrying part of this visit was when Dan 'showed' Nadine the large knife. Dan was still under the influence of drugs making him unpredictable and on edge. Nadine described intense feelings of fear, the blood draining from her face, her tongue going dry and a feeling of paralysis in her limbs. She said that her legs became numb and she was not sure she would be able to stand up and leave the flat at that point even if she had wanted to.

In supervision Nadine named her feelings in a half-joking manner which seemed to diffuse some of their strength, making them more bearable for her. We wondered whether Dan 'showing' her the knife was a veiled threat towards her or whether he was trying to communicate how he was feeling; for example, he may be frightened about her assessment and the potential loss of his partner and the baby. We discussed how it might have been helpful for Dan to know that she understood he was frightened of losing Tanya and the baby. At the time it had been very difficult for Nadine to think about responding in this way, as she was overwhelmed by her own reactions.

The reflective process helped us to recognise how feelings can be projected into us very effectively in ways which mirror what the client feels; this is what is meant by countertransference. Thinking that he may be frightened too made Nadine more sympathetic towards Dan and helped her recognise how desperate he must be feeling. However by taking her fears seriously she was also fortified in her resolve not to be placed in that kind of situation again. In supervision we were able to look at ways of managing her safety and alerting other professionals to the significant risks involved when visiting this family.

Splitting

During another supervision session Nadine described how relieved she was when her manager agreed to join her on the home visit and this had initially felt like a supportive act. However, his subsequent lateness suggested that he was more ambivalent than he had conveyed. Nadine said she experienced him as taking over during the home visit, her assessment becoming sidelined for his own agenda. It had not been helpful to talk to Tanya alone in the bedroom, as this left Nadine with Dan, exposing her to his potential violence. The manager acted protectively towards Tanya. However, Nadine thought this was at the expense of the assessment and, ironically, her own safety. The manager yawned impolitely, interrupting her questions and she wondered whether he was trying to sabotage her work. Later Nadine's feelings of vulnerability and fear during the home visit were shrugged off by the manager and she was left feeling dismissed, as if she was making a fuss about nothing. She wondered if the threat was real or all in her head. In supervision, we discussed the fact of Tanya's bruising being a demonstration of Dan's violence, validating her perception of the situation. This provided her with some relief and a confidence that she had assessed the situation thoroughly, enabling her to inform the professionals involved in the family about the risks of home visits.

In supervision Nadine was encouraged to notice how the physical arrangement during the home visit suggested a split between professionals; Nadine was left with Dan in the front room while the manager was in the bedroom with Tanya, oblivious to what was going on elsewhere. It was striking how cut-off the manager seemed to be in relation to Nadine's experience. Mirroring the family dynamics, we hypothesised that this may reflect a split-off aspect of Tanya's internal world where a large part of her mind is cut-off from her own needs and vulnerability. Each professional seems to be in touch with only one aspect of the situation, like Tanya who has contradictory sides to herself. For example, the manager is concerned with Tanya as a victim needing care and protection. Nadine is in touch with the more troubling aspects of aggression and violence in the home which Dan is acting out. However, there are hints from Dan of the violence in Tanya who, if he is telling the truth, tried to use a large knife on herself only the night before. Her destructiveness is also played out in getting drunk instead of visiting her daughter. So there are highly conflicted aspects of Tanya that are projected into those who come into contact with her, including the different professionals, who then act out the conflict with each other.

Splitting is a core defence we use to manage painful anxieties and aspects of ourselves that we would rather not acknowledge. If Tanya is only seen as a victim or a bad mother neither definition would adequately describe what was going on for her. Foster (2013), discussing the emotional deprivation of female addicts, describes the consequence of failing to address splits of this nature in clients and describes how we can collude by only seeing the good or bad aspects of the person. A failure to address all aspects of a person's experience can have devastating consequences. For example, Foster describes how a client, Mia, committed suicide partly as a result of professionals' failure to address the more disturbing aspects of her life and their collusion with her belief that she had recovered from a serious addiction problem.

Rock-a-bye baby

Following this home visit Nadine managed to observe only one further contact between Dan, Tanya, and Ayesha, which took place in a contact centre. This session was intended to be the beginning of a community-based assessment recommended after Tanya said she would not leave Dan to go into a residential unit. As it turned out, it was the last time they attended contact to see Ayesha. Nadine presented the following process recording during supervision:

> When I arrived Dan was feeding Ayesha a bottle of milk provided by the foster carer. Dan was sat leaning on a bean bag on the floor, holding Ayesha close to him and Tanya sat on the floor close to them, watching carefully. When Dan had finished feeding Ayesha he handed her over to Tanya and

began taking telephone calls, which took him out in and out of the room and gave the contact a more unsettled feel.

I asked Tanya if she thought Ayesha knew them very well, as they had missed so much contact and she responded 'she does not seem to'. Tanya made an inappropriate comment about how she was glad Ayesha was not a boy, with his penis hanging out. Tanya compared the skin tones of her own arm with Ayesha's asking whether I thought she was white. I replied that I did not know. I asked Tanya what she liked about Ayesha the most and she replied that Ayesha was 'sweet, small, cute, little and she will be a good friend to me'.

Ayesha fell asleep in the car seat and Tanya began to relax and came closer to look at her. Dan went out to make another call and Tanya began to rock Ayesha, commenting that she did not think Ayesha looked like her. She started to rock the seat quite hard and I told her to rock it more gently. Tanya said Ayesha was a 'lovely little girl' and wished she could come home with her. She stood over Ayesha and played with her arms, then picked her up out of the car seat again, jerking her on to her shoulder waking her up. While she did this she forgot to hold Ayesha's head and was insensitive to Ayesha needing to sleep.

Tanya asked where she should place Ayesha, asking on the sofa? I said there was not a sofa and I observed that she had been comfy in the car seat. Tanya said she could not get to know Ayesha in the car seat and placed her on the bean bag, commenting that Ayesha seemed to sink down into it, noting that she was going bright red and said that it was an accident. She picked her up and placed her on the floor on the changing mat and started to spin the mirrored toy around that was next to Ayesha on the floor. This had bells on the end and Tanya swung it around noisily, saying that Ayesha 'may love it very much'. She then placed a rattle in front of Ayesha's face and Tanya said 'ah, isn't she lovely'.

Tanya kept the rattle in Ayesha's face and then leaned right over her, placing her face close to Ayesha, saying 'hello'. She then swung the mirrored toy around again and while Ayesha watched it she was sick. Dan came back in just as Ayesha was sick and he wiped the mat next to her head with a cloth. As we sat watching Ayesha, Tanya began to relax again and I thought this was due to Dan's presence.

Dan picked Ayesha up and tried to feed her water and then milk again. She burped very loudly and Tanya laughed. Ayesha became very distressed despite Dan's efforts to calm her down. I noted that he became more anxious the more distressed Ayesha became and eventually I asked to take Ayesha, Dan gladly handing her over as if relieved for my help. I walked her about cuddling her into my shoulder. I noted that she was very hot and still very wet from the sick that had not been wiped off her properly earlier on. Ayesha was in a frantic state, crying for a prolonged time but I was able to calm her. This felt like a relief and although I felt terrible taking over from the parents there did not seem to be any animosity from them. When I tried to arrange contact for them afterwards they were unreachable and the assessment was brought to an end.

Supervision discussion

Nadine said that she found observing the interaction between Tanya and Ayesha excruciatingly painful and distressing. Tanya seemed to panic every time Dan left the room and she was left 'alone' with the baby. She seemed to be at a loss to know how to relate to her daughter, trying to make sense of who Ayesha was in relation to her. For example, comparing skin tones indicated the level of difficulty she had in connecting with her baby, unable to claim Ayesha as her own, or to feel as if she belonged to her. In supervision, we thought that, with hindsight, it would have been a relief for Tanya to have this anxiety named by Nadine. Tanya longs for a baby to be a friend *to her*, a reversal of the usual mother–daughter relationship. Tanya's bizarre comment about the baby's penis was disturbing, and hints at her need to use Ayesha as a receptacle for elements of her own disturbed mind (Williams, 1997).

Tanya is out of tune with Ayesha's rhythm, waking her up when she is asleep and trying to feed her when she has been fed. Tanya's spinning the mirrored toy close to Ayesha's face eventually makes her sick. This use of excitement masks the underlying pain and depression of the contact, hinting at a type of defence which has a manic quality. There are also signs of barely-suppressed hostility in Tanya's handling of Ayesha, and Nadine described how this was all the more amplified by the baby's tiny size. For example, Tanya rocked Ayesha vigorously in the car seat and picked her up by her arms, waking her from sleep. Nadine couldn't imagine that Ayesha would be safe in Tanya's care alone, even for a second. Tanya seemed to respond to Ayesha's vulnerability and complete dependency through panic and aggression, having no capacity to recognise or manage anything vulnerable in herself or in a child. Furthermore, vulnerability and helplessness seemed to provoke active hostility in her. Hostility and excitement may have been a defence against the deeper feelings of despair.

Countertransference

As Nadine read out the description of the supervised contact her voice sounded strained. She read it quickly, without pause, so that she had to be interrupted and asked to slow down. She blushed and apologised excessively for minor spelling mistakes, or she digressed from the text by adding more facts which she thought needed to be clarified. It was hard to think about the content of the session and it took another couple of goes quietly reading it through to ourselves before we could process and discuss it. It was clear how painful it was to listen to the material and how nervous Nadine was in presenting it, so much so that she seemed close to tears.

Nadine called the end of this parenting assessment her 'dirty secret' and when we explored the meaning of this she said she felt it was her fault that the assessment had ended precipitously. She fretted about whether she had done something to make the parents stay away from contact and she felt responsible for the parents' failure. She worried about what she could have done differently, or which of her actions had destroyed the potential for the baby's return home. She seemed to be experiencing feelings of guilt and shame on behalf of the parents for destroying a family. This was in stark contrast to Tanya and Dan who showed no outward signs of guilt or concern for Ayesha, appearing to be heavily defended against these painful feelings.

It seemed that Tanya and Dan were unable to grieve for the loss of their child in a straightforward way. Nadine was left with the feelings that Tanya was unable to feel. Instead, Tanya retreats from feelings into addiction and self-destructiveness, rendering herself 'mindless' in the process. Nadine experiences an unconscious fear of her own destructiveness. The monstrousness of social workers is often reinforced by the media (see Annie Hudson's (2013) critique of the media's response to the recent case where it was claimed social workers removed a child from a mother's womb). Nadine had to reconcile the painful feeling that she had torn apart a family with other extremes of emotion, as she was filled with joy and hope later when taking part in the adoption of Ayesha.

Organisational dynamics

Nadine's overall experience of her work place was as a harsh and uncaring environment. There were initiatives put in place to offer her training and support but this was fragmented and counteracted by a feeling of dysfunctional dynamics in the organisation. For example, she was particularly angry about the way this case was allocated to her at the last moment so that she had little time to prepare or make a good assessment of the mother and baby's needs. She was concerned that she was allocated a case of such complexity as an inexperienced social worker, seemingly going against the whole push towards protecting and supporting newly qualified staff. On top of these difficulties she had no consistent manager who really got to know the case along with her. The huge changes she experienced in the management left her unable to trust that she would receive help in making difficult decisions about cases. Nadine described the horror of a situation she faced early on in her job when she was instructed by a manager to visit Tanya on the same day she gave birth:

> I found that very difficult because as soon as she gave birth they told me to go down to the hospital, which I did, but I found that really, really intrusive, very intrusive, because Dan was there and it was actually quite horrible because when I went into the labour ward, she had just given birth, and so my timing was not great and unfortunately she was bleeding, because she had just had a baby and Dan was helping her with the sanitary pad and I thought, oh my god, this is too intimate and too intrusive for me and I had to stand away from them and had to tell them 'you carry on with what you are doing' and Dan took her into the bathroom and helped her, I think he helped her get a new sanitary pad and it was, it was very uncomfortable for me, I know it was really painful.

In supervision we attempted to look at how we thought the organisation was acting in this situation. We wondered about the level of complexity of the work expected from a newly qualified member of staff. From discussions with Tanya it appeared to be an agency that could not meet the needs of its newest members, with vulnerability being abused in the worker and mother alike. Nadine said she could not help feeling that if she were more experienced, or had better line management support, she may have made different decisions about Tanya and Ayesha's care – perhaps pushing for a mother and baby foster placement where both their needs for care could be met and a fuller assessment made. She believed there was more emphasis on the control aspect of the work than the care element.

From Nadine's descriptions and the supervisor's initial strong response to the projection that she was being exploited and abused, we turned a distracted and somewhat neglectful organisation into an actively abusive one in our minds. We were left wondering whether we had been caught up with our own projections into the organisation or indeed whether they were the supervisor's own projections. Was this an accurate depiction of the organisation? After all, this was the same local authority that had commissioned the supervision, perhaps as a way of ameliorating the inherent failures in the system.

Abuser/abused

Looking at the countertransference response as the pull towards the enactment of sado-masochistic dynamics we could begin to hypothesise about the state of Tanya's internal world. The psychoanalyst Jane Milton (1994) describes how difficult it is to work with women who have been abused as there is constant pressure to enact perverse internal object relationships. It is difficult to consider someone as vulnerable as Tanya, an obvious victim of horrendous abuse, as a potential perpetrator of abuse. As professionals, we can struggle to view the victim as perpetrator and we can endlessly take sides, blaming one parent or the other for being the 'baddie'. This prevents us from seeing the function each individual has for the other in the couple as a whole. Milton reminds us that being 'the abused' is often inextricably linked with being 'the abuser'. She explains that this is because 'masochism involves the accompanying projection of sadism, forcing the other to be the helpless witness of suffering in which they are supposed to be implicated' (Milton, 1994: 243).

Regarding the treatment of sexually abused women, Milton writes;

> Sympathetic attention to the person who has been a helpless victim is essential. At the same time it is vital to address what is perhaps the most serious aspect of the victim's plight; her corruption in childhood via excessive stimulation of her own hatred and destructiveness, which becomes erotised, and her identification with the aggressor, often as a means of psychic survival. A one-sided 'idealisation' of the victim aspect, although very tempting, may do such

patients (and ultimately the next generation of in the cycle of abuse and neglect), a great disservice.

(Milton, 1994: 243)

Foster describes how the deprivation of female drug addicts gets repeated by a system of care whereby organisations become punitive and punishing like the harsh internal world of the client (2013: 87). Munro touches on organisational dynamics and the need for support in her review commenting that:

> Being exposed to the powerful and often negative emotions found in child protection work comes at a personal cost. If the work environment does not help support workers and debrief them after particularly traumatic experiences, then it increases the risk of burnout which, in the human services, has been defined in terms of three dimensions: emotional exhaustion, depersonalisation (or cynicism), and reduced personal accomplishment.

(Munro, 2011)

Disappointment and the failure of omnipotence – Anna Harvey

> The boy stood on the burning deck
> Whence all but he had fled;
> The flame that lit the battle's wreck
> Shone round him o'er the dead.
> Yet beautiful and bright he stood,
> As born to rule the storm –
> A creature of heroic blood,
> A proud, though child-like form.
> (Casabianca, Hemans, 1826)

Child protection social workers experience the most extraordinary of circumstances while helping those 'in need' with their lives. They encounter highly pressurised situations where levels of responsibility are huge. Like the burning deck, the work is dangerous, emotionally demanding, intense and potentially traumatising. It can feel like you are the last resort, particularly when it comes to the most difficult of situations, such as a child protection investigation or removing children from their parents. Social workers are expected to make clear, well thought-through, rational decisions whilst under enormous pressure. This is a pressure arising from both external and internal sources. In some cases the decisions social workers make will affect the parent and child for the rest of their lives. In addition to this huge level of responsibility, social workers need to process levels of complexity about risk and decipher what is in the best interests of a child. These levels of complexity are hard to countenance by the lay person.

Unlike the child in the poem, social workers are of course adults with adult capacities, acting within wider professional systems which support their decision making. However, social workers' adult capacities and judgement can be destabilised by the emotional factors or unconscious processes involved in child protection work. Unconscious processes include: the impact of infantile projections of an emotionally deprived part of the parent or child which the worker can become projectively identified with; a pressure to act in a certain way by the parent through overt or covert hostility, or the pressure to think in the same way as the parent; resentments between social worker and line manager leading to problems in the organisation being acted out on the family. Under these circumstances it is little wonder that decisions for children can go wrong. It is our responsibility to understand the emotional and unconscious pressures, so that social workers can think about their emotional experiences and make well-thought-through decisions which are not just responses to unconscious factors.

Unlike the child who stood on the burning deck social workers do not work in isolation. They have a manager and they are part of a team and inter-professional system. However, the pressure to act and take the lead in making the most serious of decisions usually falls to the judgement of the individual social worker. This will be in dialogue with their manager and will be based on their observations and their perceived effectiveness of their intervention with the family. If the relationship between the social worker and manager is strained and no true reflection which involves *thinking* and *feeling* takes place then decisions can be poorly thought-through, reactionary and precipitous, reflecting the unconscious dynamics between the parties rather than what is in the best interests of the child. If the social worker is not supported properly by their organisation or even a social policy context that is cognisant of the difficulty of the primary task (assessing whether child abuse has occurred), then they are vulnerable psychologically, just like children, to the traumatising effects of the cases.

The poem above is ambiguous but it may also describe an omnipotent, heroic fantasy of a child who has the belief that he can stop a burning ship all by himself. I would suggest that social workers, their organisations, policy contexts and developments in training and education often collude with a similar idea, where social workers, child-like in their preparedness for the psychological pressures of the task, are thrust prematurely into quite challenging and complex child protection work. They are even expected to take up leadership roles prematurely, before really knowing what the work entails.

The precociousness implicit in educational programmes such as Frontline and Step Up to Social Work, where only the best and brightest of graduates will be chosen to become the social workers of our futures (and by implication resolve all of the recruitment and retention problems) hints at the fantasy of the heroic. However, in my own experience of providing reflective supervision to Newly Qualified Social Workers (NQSW) from the Step-Up and Frontline programmes it is often the brightest who realise the impossibility of the task first and are therefore the first to leave. Anecdotally, in one year of providing reflective supervision to nine Step Up NQSWs, five left, travelling abroad or moving into the voluntary sector. Despite huge investment by the organisation in the Step Up students' training, education, supervision and then post-qualifying training, most felt justified in leaving. Some expressed a feeling of betrayal by the local authority who they complained had not 'lived up to its end of the bargain'. They were disappointed with the levels of support despite seeming to be extensive. However, this disappointing feeling may have related more realistically to the kinds of experiences where they were disappointed with their ability to effect change in certain cases. Or, in one case, a realisation of the emotional deprivation and harm the looked after children on their caseload had experienced.

For example, Roger, a young Asian, male social worker was a highly energetic, proactive and engaged newly qualified worker. He brought a case to supervision involving four young children in foster care. Their mother had missed a number of recent contact sessions, to the children's huge disappointment, a disappointment that the mother did not face but which the social worker did. The social worker explained that he had to help the children to understand why she wasn't coming. This was something the older children wearily understood but the disappointment for the youngest made him feel very angry with the mother and sad for the children. They were in care due to their mother having a serious alcohol problem, which had brought them to social services' attention over many years. It was very unlikely that the mother would engage in any treatment programme where change would occur. Therefore, the children were unlikely to return to her care. Their foster care situation had just deteriorated. The male foster carer had suddenly discovered he had cancer of the liver. This had spread around his body and he died shockingly quickly over a two-week period. The children saw their own respective fathers, but none of their fathers were in a position to care for them, as they either lived with new partners and children or had addiction problems themselves.

Roger complained in supervision about 'the managers' and their decision making. He was of the strong opinion that the children had not been protected from harm in the past, as they had been accommodated only to be returned home again. Now he was picking up the pieces again after things had broken down and they had come into care. He inferred that he could make much better decisions and felt passionately about the children. He thought they should move immediately and a new long-term carer should be found.

Towards the middle of supervision Roger admitted to me that he had an interview for a neighbouring borough. I was familiar with disgruntled social workers leaving to work in this local authority, only to hear later on that they had moved again. Because I had built up a good relationship with Roger he began to reveal that the real reason he wanted to move local authorities was that he didn't want to work with long-term cases again. He would only work in a referral and assessment team in the future, somewhere he said he would have limited engagement with the family. The case would be open for a short time before he could pass it on. On deeper discussion, he revealed that he had found working with the four children extremely painful. He could not see a good outcome for them. He was angry at their mother for missing contact. The younger children had started to turn away from him, angry at his failure to return them home to their mother. Despite the supervision perhaps getting to the heart of the matter, Roger was offered a new job at a higher pay scale. He moved into the Referral and Assessment Team in the neighbouring local authority.

Conclusion

Social workers, alongside certain social intervention programmes (such as the Troubled Families Programme), are expected to act heroically, to bring about the change that will prevent harm to the child even if that means sacrificing their own psychological and emotional well-being. We can also see this fantasy implicit in public outcries when an awareness of a child's death breaks into the public consciousness. Social workers are blamed as they are expected to be omniscient and able to prevent the tragedy from occurring in the first place. This is an omnipotent fantasy which mirrors the unconscious dynamics in abusive or ill families where children can be looked to unconsciously by the parents to resolve intractable problems in themselves.

There has been little research into the enormity of the emotional pressures on complex child protection work, and the implications of unconscious processes on decision making. Fortunately, there have been developments in this area, for example in the important research being undertaken by Harry Ferguson (2016), and the chapters by Charlotte Noyes and Fiona Henderson in the present volume. However, generally the policy makers, organisation and professional system all tend to underestimate the emotional impact of this kind of work on the social worker. There is a culture of machismo, a denial of vulnerability, and a turning away from a full acknowledgement of the complexity and disturbing nature of the primary task. The individualising nature of case work leaves social workers susceptible to being drawn into unconscious dynamics projected from the parent, usually at the expense of the child. Or social workers experience projective identification with the emotional deprivation in the child. When overwhelmed by the parents' needs arising from early emotional deprivation and neglect, it is nearly impossible to keep the parent–child dyad in mind without the right kind of help. When identified with the child's pain, social workers may find themselves becoming stuck, unable to act decisively, or they may begin to distance themselves from the work by finding new opportunities elsewhere.

However, the social worker can be contained by a supportive framework, their organisation, and a sensitive attendance to the emotional and unconscious factors involved in the work by their supervisor. Adult capacities can be reinstated through reflective supervision and decisions reached which keep the parent–child dyad in mind. This will promote well-thought-through decisions which are made in a collaborative and supportive atmosphere. This requires a policy context fully cognisant of the complexity and psychological dangerousness of the primary task. Developing the capacity for deep reflexivity takes time and experience over years. We should indeed attract the best and brightest into the profession, but we should not then expect them to be able to cope psychologically with the more extreme forms of abuse and neglect (I was introduced to child protection work over years). Neither should we look to them to be a quick fix for the inherent problems in the child protection system.

The case study illustrates the dynamic tensions at work during a home visit and contact session, and encapsulates the highly disturbing nature of social work practice. This is work which stirs the most basic anxieties in all of us: anxieties about vulnerability, helplessness and about our potential to do harm. Psychoanalytic theory is uniquely placed to account for these complexities of human nature and to help workers understand their emotional responses to this difficult work. Social workers have to be especially attuned to the potential for emotional disturbance and hostility in parents and to be aware of destructive forces governing behaviour, especially those with underlying mental illness or personality disturbance.

Being in contact with this kind of disturbance on a regular basis can be extremely unsettling, affecting our sense of well-being and sometimes our personal lives, and making it harder to be an effective resource for our clients. Concepts such as projective identification can help us understand how cases 'get under our skin' to the extent that they do. It is important to notice and make sense of projective processes to lessen the chance of becoming burned-out or resentful in our approach to the work. Reflective supervision in individual or group format provides an opportunity to consider case material in detail and depth, including the ways in which we are affected by our clients. Reflective supervision guided by a psychoanalytic framework provides a sophisticated model of containment that takes account of both conscious and unconscious factors in drawing together an understanding of a case. If the social worker can be better contained in their involvement with a case then they will be in a stronger position to offer the kind of containment that our clients desperately need.

Editors' afterword

This chapter illustrates how the dynamics of malfunctioning families can become enacted among the staff of a social services department. The conflict between Tanya and Dan, the clients, is enacted by Nadine, a newly qualified social worker, and her manager. The manager identifies with Dan, seeing him as the responsible parent, and using his position to dismiss Nadine's point of view. Meanwhile in another room and out of sight, Dan subtly uses a knife to intimidate Nadine. The feelings of guilt and inadequacy that Dan and Tanya might feel for not managing their baby are projected into Nadine, who feels she should be able to keep this family together. Ironically, baby Ayesha is getting a better deal than her mother, who was left in an abusive family. It is interesting that Tanya's treatment of her baby amounts to abuse. One wonders what her own experience was as a baby.

Anna Harvey draws attention to the way in which the bright 'fast track' young social workers are supposed to 'put right' the problems in the child protection system. One problem that cannot be 'solved' is the emotional experience of taking a baby away from its mother. Melanie Klein has shown that it is part of normal development for a small child to want to rob its mother of her babies. This is a normal unconscious phantasy, which usually remains as a phantasy. A social worker, when asked to turn this phantasy into a reality, can find this extremely disturbing. One social worker told us that she had never forgotten the first baby she took into care thirty years previously.

References

Bower, M. (2003) Broken and twisted. *Journal of Social Work Practice* 17(2), 143–151.

Bower, M. (2005) Psychoanalytic theories for social work practice. In: Bower, M. (ed.) *Psychoanalytic Theory for Social Work Practice – Thinking Under Fire*. London: Routledge.

Britton, R. (2005) Re-enactment as an unwitting professional response to family dynamics. In: Bower, M. (ed.) *Psychoanalytic Theory for Social Work Practice – Thinking Under Fire*. London: Routledge.

Ferguson, H. (2016) How children become invisible in child protection work. *British Journal of Social Work* 0, 1–18.

Foster, A. (2013) The deprivation of female drug addicts. In: Bower, M., Hale, R. and Wood, H. (eds) *Addictive States of Mind*. London: Karnac.

Hudson, A. (2013) *The Guardian*, 10 December.

Milton, J. (1994) Abuser and abused: perverse solutions following childhood abuse. *Psychoanalytic Psychotherapy* 8(3), 243–255.

Munro, E. (2011) *The Munro Review of Child Protection: Final Report. A Child Centred System.* London: UK Government.

Rustin, M. and Bradley, J. (2008) *Work Discussion. Learning from Reflective Practice in Work with Children and Families*. London: Karnac.

Williams, G. (1997) Reversal of the container/contained relationship. In: *Internal Landscapes and Foreign Bodies. Eating Disorders and Other Pathologies*. London: Karnac, pp. 103–114.

6

IDENTIFYING 'BLIND SPOTS' WHEN MOVING CHILDREN FROM FOSTER CARE INTO ADOPTION

Lynne Cudmore and Sophie Boswell

The paediatrician and psychoanalyst Donald Winnicott drew attention to the long-term impact of early separations, describing the experience as traumatic:

> Trauma means the breaking of the continuity of the line of an individual's existence. It is only on a continuity of existing that the sense of self, of feeling real, and of being, can eventually be established as a feature of the individual personality.

> *(Winnicott, 1986)*

Winnicott believed that the quality of the environment around the child is crucial in helping them to manage any such 'breaks in continuity'. In his view, the extent of the trauma suffered depends on whether the adults looking after the child are able to remain sensitive and attuned to the disruption and loss that the child is experiencing. In this chapter we will be exploring the break in continuity experienced by children when they become adopted, and the ways in which the adults around them struggle to remain attuned to their emotional experience, and particularly to the experience of loss during this transition.

Adoption offers huge long-term gains for children, but leaving the care of their previous home also involves a major loss. Many adopted children, especially those under three years old, will have lived with their foster carer for most of their lives, so that she has become their 'psychological mother' (Robertson and Robertson, 1989). Time spent with birth parents is likely to have been unstable, or characterised by neglect or abuse. So it is the foster carer and her family who have provided the only consistent and safe parenting these children have known. In spite of this, the significance of the foster carer relationship for the child's emotional development is often forgotten when the focus falls on the other two parties in the adoption 'triangle', the birth parents and the adopters.

The best environment for children to feel safe enough to settle into their new family and build up a feeling of trust and safety with their adoptive parents will be one in which the adults around them recognise that they are likely to be experiencing a major loss, and are able to support them emotionally by remaining attuned to what this loss means for them. However, with the intensity of feelings stirred up – in the foster carers, the adopters and the social workers – this can be exceptionally hard to do. It is a highly complex emotional task for everyone involved to hold in mind the loss of a meaningful relationship while nurturing a new one.

While working alongside social workers in the field of fostering and adoption, we became concerned about how quickly children were being moved, and how little contact there was with foster carers afterwards. Our social work colleagues seemed unclear about the reasons why moves were carried out so quickly and there was confusion about when and indeed whether it was helpful for the child to see the foster carer again. Our own experience of helping to support these transitions gave us first-hand experience of what an emotionally charged time it was for all the adults involved, and how difficult it was to raise awareness of the child's loss in the midst of this anxiety without being seen as 'spoiling' the positive feelings about the adoption.

We realised how little guidance there was for understanding this huge transition in a child's life; and that holding in mind the array of emotional experiences for the child was often made more difficult as children rarely expressed feelings of anger or distress during the move, either in words or through their behaviour. A preliminary literature review identified an absence of research into this area. Although there is a huge amount of research examining the impact of contact between adopted children and their birth families, we could find almost nothing on contact with foster carers after adoption.

In order to gauge current practices in the field we carried out an audit of our own agency and an informal survey of adoption agencies across the UK, collecting data on their policies regarding speed of move and contact with carers post adoption, and what they understood to be the rationale behind them. The responses showed that children are usually moved within seven to fourteen days of meeting their new parents and once moved will generally not see their foster carer again for at least three months, often longer, and that some will never see her again. Younger children and babies tend to be moved more quickly. Contradicting reasons were given about contact. Some agencies told us that older children with a deeper attachment to their foster carer needed slightly earlier contact; others cited a strong attachment to the foster carer as a reason to *avoid* contact after the move for fear of unsettling the child.

Our research project

Joining forces with three social workers in the adoption team, we set up a small, qualitative research project to explore what factors might be driving current procedures in this area. As a research methodology we chose to use Interpretational Phenomenological Analysis (IPA) as it aims 'to understand lived experience and how participants themselves make sense of their experiences' (Smith, 2009). We were not gauging the emotional experience of each child during their move, but trying to understand what was informing the adults' decision-making process at different stages of the process. IPA, with its use of interviews and close analysis, allowed us to explore deeply the ways in which the key players experienced this very complex period of time and how their own responses and feelings affected the decisions they made on behalf of the children.

We chose four relatively recent cases involving five children, two of whom were siblings. As it happened, four of the children chosen were between nine and fourteen months old when they moved, and the fifth was two years old. It seemed that all of the adoptions were felt to have gone relatively smoothly. We had not intended to restrict ourselves to younger children or to smooth transitions, and initially this seemed to present a problem. However, we increasingly came to believe that one of the key questions we were trying to answer was how adults were able to make sense of the children's reactions to the transition. This emerged as particularly complex with children who were pre-verbal or less able to show their feelings. Babies and younger children tended to be described as less 'problematic', and therefore less attention was generally given to their emotional state. We realised that it was important to us that we should draw attention to this, and to question whether a young child or baby who does not cry or show major signs of upset should really be taken as one who is 'fine'; and, more generally, for any age group, we wanted to question whether a 'smooth' transition should really be considered the most desirable kind.

As one might expect, all of the children had already experienced turbulence prior to adoption. One was a relinquished baby who had been with her foster carer from birth. Another had been taken into care after spending his first few weeks in hospital suffering from foetal alcohol syndrome. One child had experienced severe neglect in her parents' care for her first few weeks before being placed with her carer. Another had been removed in traumatic circumstances when her parents were discovered to be physically abusing her older siblings. The last child, her younger brother, had been placed with one first foster carer at birth, but after a few months had been moved to join his sister in her placement, prior to their being adopted together, thus experiencing two moves within his first year of life.

The interviews

We carried out semi-structured interviews with foster carers, adopters and at least two members of the social work team around each case (this was usually the child's social worker, the foster carer's support worker and/or adopters' social worker). Where there was a couple we invited both members, and although the foster carers' partners chose not to take part, all of the adopters did. Three of the foster carers were highly experienced, one was moving a baby for the first time. One of the adoptive couples had already adopted a child. Wherever possible each interview was carried out by a child psychotherapist and a social worker. Interview questions were kept brief and were designed to encourage participants to tell their story in their own way.

As we analysed the data from our interviews, in great detail, it quickly became clear that the child's relationship with their foster carer, and possible feelings about losing her, took up different spaces in people's minds, and in fact altered significantly over different phases of the transition. We have attempted to trace this thread, looking at how the child's relationship to their carer was perceived in people's minds before, during and after the move.

Early days: 'It was like I'd given birth to her'

We looked first at the period before the formal 'introductions meeting', where the network meets for the first time to make plans for the move. During this stage all of the adults were mindful of the emotional significance of the relationship between the child and the carer. Foster carers spoke with great warmth about the child within their family: the language was full of words such as 'love', 'adored', 'part of the family', 'belonged', 'like my own baby'.

FOSTER CARER (FC): I don't think they realise you've had her from a baby, and you end up loving them ... You raise them like yours, you care for them like your own kids

FC: It was like I'd given birth to her

Most foster carers were not only very in-tune with how much they mattered to the child, but also acutely aware of these children's troubled backgrounds, how vulnerable this made them to separations:

FC: Even short separations matter for babies, their emotions would be all over the place and for me to go off ... I just couldn't do it.

The adopters also spoke warmly about the importance of this early period in the children's lives, and of the bond between child and carer. Many of them expressed gratitude for the way in which the child had been cared for and loved.

ADOPTIVE PARENT (AP): They adored her, they really did. We could see that she was part of a very lovely family.

Adopters felt that having a strong attachment to their foster carer was very important for the child's emotional development. One adoptive parent expressed concern that her child may not have been passionately attached to her foster carer, and that this might have an impact on her capacity to make future attachments. Another couple were worried that their adopted son had shown no overt distress when having to change foster carers at nine months old. The importance of these early attachments was very strong in the adults' minds. There was also a depth of emotion attributed to these children so that they came across as having their feelings understood and responded to by carers and prospective adopters alike.

Planning stage: 'Not my baby'

From the introductions meeting onwards, we were struck by how the tone of all of the adults changed, so that the less intimate language of procedures and plans began to dominate. The foster carer, in her own and other people's eyes, became less of a 'mother' and more of a professional with a job to do. As the focus shifted to making plans for the introductory visits, it seemed more difficult to focus on the emotional complexity of the child's experience during this upheaval in their lives. Although a great deal of attention was given to the need for continuity of routine – food, toys, bedtime arrangements – it seemed much harder for the adults to remain fully in touch with the children's emotional state and the fact that it was a loved person that they would be losing.

Talking about the lead-up to the move, it was clear that foster carers were processing some very painful feelings and many of them were explicit about how giving in to these feelings was incompatible with retaining a professional stance. Their language became more procedural, less personal. The child was no longer a beloved member of their family but a prospective member of someone else's. They no longer felt they had the right to feel passionate about the child, and the more experienced carers described how they had to 'stand back' emotionally from the child as a prelude to 'letting them go'. The most common reason given for this 'standing back' was the need to support the adopters in their role as new parents. The foster carers revealed an acute sensitivity to the feelings of the adopters, their need to feel empowered as parents and an awareness of how threatened or undermined they could feel if the carer were to bring attention to the bond between carer and child:

FC: You have to be very careful what you say to an adopter, you don't want to come across as if, 'You have taken my child', because this has never been my child. People say, 'How can you give her?' Well she's not mine to give away, she's never been mine you know, I'm looking after her. So saying to an adopter, 'I'm really going to miss her and I don't know what I'll do without her and it'll absolutely break my heart' – that's not helpful.

This attitude was widely shared. Social workers also spoke about the need for the foster carer to remain 'professional' and not let her emotions spill out, to protect adoptive parents from being burdened with the child's attachment and impending loss. Adopters, although highly aware of the personal pain the foster carers were experiencing, were grateful to them for keeping it to themselves. Already in a state of high anxiety, they felt they could not have coped with the foster carer bombarding them with her own feelings of loss, or with the level of attachment between herself and the child. One couple told us about a previous adoption where a foster carer had confided in them about how much the child was going to miss her, and they had been deeply shocked, describing this as unprofessional and undermining. In this context it is not surprising that adopters felt grateful to the network for guiding them through the process in an efficient and practical way, avoiding a flood of emotions.

AP: It's probably very good to focus on the practicalities, and to take all the emotion out of it because the week of transitions was going to be pretty emotional all round, so it was good to have a sort of business-like approach to it all, and just focus on the practicalities.

One of the carers, who was moving a baby for the first time, was troubled by the way that the network appeared to disapprove of her expressing her sad feelings.

FC: It doesn't give you any time to think and re-adjust. I found it difficult. Maybe I'm just – you know, there's love involved.

Some of the adopters also voiced ambivalence about how little room was given for the emotions involved, even though it felt helpful at the time:

AP: That [the planning meeting] was an empty sort of debate ... it was processed and there was nothing else in terms of the emotional aspect that was talked about.

With so much preoccupation with how the adults were managing their feelings, it seemed difficult for anyone to fully keep in mind what might be going on for the children. In thinking about plans for contact after adoption, most of the interviewees spoke of this as being done either for the sake of the foster carers, who would be missing the children, or for the sake of the adopters who might like some support from the carers.

FC: I think what's discussed at the meetings is oh yeah the carer is, I suppose, for want of a better word is entitled to see the child a few months after they've left ... You wouldn't really want to see the child before three months, you've got to give the child that ...
INTERVIEWER (I): Is that your view, or is that what you've heard?
FC: No, but that's the initial offer you would get, put it that way, you would get an offer of maybe one visit after the child's gone.

What seemed more absent from people's minds at this stage was the capacity to imagine what it might mean for the child to see their carer again after the move, or what it might feel like *not* to see her.

Moving homes: 'It wasn't a big deal'

It was during the actual move that we felt adults struggled the most to remain open to what was happening for the child emotionally. All of the children were moved from their foster carers' to their adopters' home in a period of between seven and ten days, in line with the national average. The adults spoke of this as a kind of 'rollercoaster', quite overwhelming and exhausting, but they believed that it was better like this, rather than 'dragging things out'.

The children were described as surprisingly compliant, showing little outward sign of emotional turmoil. The adopters and carers – and social workers too – admitted feeling anxious about a child becoming openly distressed, and put great effort into minimising the disruption for the children. There was a huge sense of relief when the children did not show distress during the move. Although every-one had been aware of how deeply attached these children were to their carers, at this stage there was no concern expressed when children appeared not to be upset by being separated from them. In fact, all the upset feelings were seen as residing in the adults, while the children were frequently described as 'fine':

FC: From the child's point of view it wasn't a big deal. She was quite relaxed and happy. She had only had one carer, me, and she was moving to another.

I: You mean, you could tell she was managing it at the time?

FC: The attachment was just going to be transferred straight over and it did go straight over.

Foster carers and social workers often cited this idea that a child who has had a stable attachment to one carer will be able to attach more quickly to a new one, but this seemed to obscure the knowledge that there was still a huge loss involved.

Adopters, perhaps taking their cue from the foster carers, also tended to be relieved to find that the child appeared to be basically all right, not appearing to be missing their foster carer, while all too aware of the loss and separation experienced by the foster carer and her family while the child was being moved:

ADOPTIVE MOTHER (AM): I don't know, the real challenge for them was always to remember that she is going to be leaving them one day. And throughout the transition week you could see the emotion.

ADOPTIVE FATHER: They were finding it really really difficult …

AM: I think you know she [foster carer] could steel herself but he [carer's husband] was just totally besotted with the baby and I think he found it incredibly difficult … I think it was incredibly difficult.

The moment of final separation was described by everyone as emotionally intense, and even the most experienced foster carers could not completely hide their feelings. However the children were still described as fine. In the following excerpt, the foster carer spoke about the moment of saying goodbye for the last time:

FC: There was a bit of tears too.
I: From you and them?
FC: And them, yes.
I: Both of them?
FC: No, not from the children, because they were used to that period, going and coming back.
I: Oh. All the adults?
FC: The adults. [laughs] They said, 'Oh we're taking the children from you' and saying 'We're Mum and Dad now, we'll look after them for the rest of their lives'.
I: Very emotional. But do you think the children were just, 'We're off "bye bye!"'?
FC: The children said, 'Bye mummy, bye, bye! ... I can see the car going.' [cries]

The language used to describe the children here was much less rich or emotionally complex than it had been when describing their life and their feelings prior to the transition; in fact, they came across as emotionally thin and lacking deep feelings.

AP: She was fine, and she quite enjoyed her new high chair and stuff, so you know she was. Yeah it worked brilliantly, we just felt so incredibly fortunate because it just went so smoothly.

We found that quite often we needed to ask follow-up questions to guide interviewees back to the children's experience, as this quite often got lost.

I: Can we go back a little bit, how was [the child] during that week?
AM: He was fine – he was never clingy, he never started screaming Mummy or asking for [his carer] when he was there.

When there were flickers of being in touch with something happening at a deeper level for the child during the separation, this came across as very painful for foster carers, who tended to shy away from lingering on this.

FC: The day he left we stood there and he saw my tears and [my husband] said, 'Look at him, looking at you'.
I: Did he look sad himself?
FC: Well, he did. It's almost for a second he looked and the face changed ... now I look back at the photo ... he has this face as if it's a recognition, it's a recognition of me you know? And you can see it in the photograph. He all of a sudden had this look, it wasn't smiling, not a smiley look, and I think he was

probably, you know … A very knowing look. But still happy for me to pass him over. There was no clinging to take me back like that. He went over to them well.

The adults derived comfort from the fact that the move had gone 'smoothly' and the child didn't 'cling'. This appeared to be a huge relief, indicating that the move had gone well.

After the move: 'Let sleeping dogs lie'

After the heightened anxiety and tension described during the actual move, the foster carers, once alone, spoke of a sudden outpouring of suppressed grief and emotion. They described the aftermath of losing the child on a personal level, very much like bereavement.

FC: I cried for days when she left.

In contrast, almost all of the foster carers told us that they did not imagine the child would be missing them. Adopters also tended to describe the emotions of the children as hard to read or as apparently quite bland, as if they were hardly affected at all – with one exception, a baby who cried for six weeks, would not be put down and clung to her adoptive mother, causing a lot of concern, before eventually settling down. More typical was this sort of account:

AP: I thought they'd wake up in the morning and be crying because they wouldn't know where they were but they were both standing up in their cots smiling at us and I thought this is a fluke. But they never ever cried, it was lovely.

There seemed to be a sense of great relief after the move that the children were not showing open distress or crying for their foster carers.

Contact between child and carer

Adoptive parents were mostly left to make the final decision about when – or whether – the child had contact with their foster carer, and most described being unsure about what was best for the child. They found it hard to judge whether or not the child wanted to see their carer, and in the light of the child appearing to be fine, they feared that seeing the foster carer might disturb the new attachment, unsettle the child's equilibrium, 'rock the boat'. In the event, one set of adopters delayed the first contact for about six months; another family arranged a one-off contact after three months; and another family did not pursue contact at all. The one adopter who kept up contact with the foster carer described this as for her own sake rather than for the child's.

The foster carers were the most vocal about the need for a gap of several months prior to contact happening. Most expressed a fear of intruding, forcing themselves in and stirring up distress for the new family. They used expressions like 'stepping on the adopters' toes', 'standing between' the child and the new parents, not knowing when they were not wanted, or burdening the happy family with their own feelings of grief.

FC: So I leave it with them to contact me, it's entirely up to them and I'm not going to say that they're terrible people cos they haven't, cos they're dealing with their emotions with their new child, do they really have to worry about yours at the same time?

Again, all feelings of missing, of pining to see a lost person, are seen to reside with the carer and her family alone – not the child. As on the whole the children appeared to be fine, not showing signs of registering their loss, the prospect of a too-early contact with the carer raised fears of an uncontained outpouring of distress, images of a clinging, sobbing child. This was something that was felt to be unfair on the child and highly undermining and painful for the adopters and foster carers.

FC: I mean I would hate to go and visit a child and the child is screaming and clinging on to me. I'd be horrified that I'd do that to a child, it means you've gone there too soon, it shouldn't be happening. Cos I think if you're standing in the middle of the child and the couple or the child and the other person, the child gets very confused and I think that you're taking that away from … Am I making it too complicated?

For those who decided to pursue contact some months down the line, both adopters and foster carers found it reassuring if the child appeared to have forgotten the carer.

FC: What I want to do is I want to go and visit that child and that child looks at me and goes, 'Hmm, I think I know you, but I want my Mum,' and then I go, 'Yes!' You know what I mean? My job's done.

I: Do you want to go back sort of when they're not missing you any more?

FC: Yeah. Maybe I'm protecting myself, I don't know.

It was hard to untangle exactly whose feelings were being protected by this delay in contact, but it seemed to provide a retreat from having to witness unbearable displays of loss or grief. Among the adults, including social workers, there was a widely held belief that it was better, as one adoptive parent put it, to 'let sleeping dogs lie'. The aim seemed to be to help the child to 'forget' as quickly as possible, hoping that 'out of sight' might mean 'out of mind'.

Overall, there seemed to be a shared belief among adopters, foster carers and social workers that old attachments needed to be forgotten about before new ones could be made, leaving any underlying grief to subside as quickly and quietly as possible.

Analysis: the blind spot

Our interviews threw up a rich and complex set of data, and gave us a very vivid picture of what was a highly complex, emotionally intense period for everyone concerned. Our interviewees showed a clear capacity for sensitivity, warmth, thoughtfulness and concern for the children they spoke about and for each other. However, at the actual point of making decisions about how quickly the child was going to move, during the move itself and in the period immediately afterwards, we felt that there was a heightened state of anxiety among the adults that created a sort of collective 'blind spot', hampering their capacity to retain the thoughtful, reflective state of mind essential to remaining in touch with what a young child might be feeling.

Foster carers and adopters are all faced with a massive task in trying to pick their way through a maelstrom of emotions, the pain of loss and the excitement of becoming parents, with very little guidance available about what might be happening for the child. We believe that the following factors contributed:

- It was difficult to square the happiness of adoption with the sadness of loss.
- People did not want to undermine adopters or 'spoil' the positive side of adoption by bringing attention to loss or to the child's former attachments.
- Adults were nervous about upsetting or confusing the child, raking up distress that was better hidden, hoping that out of sight meant out of mind (Robertson and Robertson, 1989).
- Foster carers found the idea of the child missing them very painful, and possibly preferred not to dwell on it.
- Faced with pre-verbal or uncommunicative children, no one felt confident or informed enough to explore what might be happening behind the child's apparent lack of emotion at losing their carer.
- The adults in general appeared to find the pain of the child's loss hard to keep in mind, retreating into a kind of 'organisational defence' (Menzies Lyth, 1988) which replaced emotional pain with practicalities and procedures.
- No one really knew what to do in the light of insufficient research/evidence so deferred to a 'the way we've always done it' approach.

Our knowledge base on the making and breaking of attachments

Our research has led us to identify a gap between our collective knowledge base, informed by a basic understanding of attachment and loss, and the way that children are currently moved from foster carer into adoptive families. Our collective knowledge base, a combination of theory, practice and accumulated experience, could be summarised in the following terms:

1. Losing a parent figure in childhood is traumatic at whatever age it happens but particularly in the first three to four years of life (Bowlby, 1980; Rutter,

1971; Breier et al, 1988; Winnicott, 1986). Children who have had a good first attachment may well be better able to form new attachments in time, but their pain and loss will be just as profound.

2. Children experiencing such a loss – particularly those who have already lost attachment figures, and even more for those who been exposed to parental neglect or mistreatment – are likely to experience acute feelings of confusion, mistrust, fear and a sense of abandonment. (Hindle and Schuman, 2008; Burnell et al., 2009; Sinclair et al., 2005).

3. How the loss is planned for and managed, how gentle or how abrupt the separation is and how much emotional support and understanding is given to the child at this time are all crucial factors in deciding how traumatic this loss may be and how well the child can recover from it. (Breier et al, 1988; Winnicott, 2004; Aldgate and Simmonds, 1988).

4. As long as it is handled sensitively, the ongoing presence of an existing attachment figure, remaining available and continuing to have a supportive role, can reassure and help children rather than adding to their confusion; and it can also remove the trauma of sudden and unaccountable loss (Bowlby, 1980; Robertson and Robertson, 1989).

5. The grieving process, which includes the expression of distress and anger, is psychologically crucial if the child is to recover from significant loses and go on to make deep and trusting relationships. (Freud, 1917; Klein, 1940; Bowlby, 1980; Fahlberg, 1994; Lanyado, 2003; Hindle and Shulman, 2008). As Vera Fahlberg puts it, 'Unresolved grief interferes with forming new attachments and the more abrupt the loss the harder it is to complete the grieving process' (Fahlberg, 1994).

6. As adults it is hard to witness the rawness of a child's suffering. This is true even in an ordinary setting, let alone in situations of such profound loss. Our capacity to be emotionally attuned and responsive to children suffering from loss will have a big impact on their capacity to mourn and to recover and to trust in new relationships. Conversely, adults who cannot bear the children's pain can become cut off themselves and unwittingly send out a message that the children's feelings are unwanted. Although planning carefully to minimise the pain of a move is crucial, we have to be careful not to be lulled into believing that with enough continuity and planning the pain of loss can not only be minimised but avoided altogether. (Fahlberg, 1994; Sinclair et al., 2005; Romaine et al., 2007; Sellick et al., 2004; Dozier, 2007; Robertson and Robertson, 1989).

7. Children react to loss in a variety of ways and do not always show their distress overtly. Even in infancy children who are already vulnerable because of early neglect, abuse or separations are particularly prone to defend themselves by cutting themselves off from their emotional state, becoming outwardly compliant and apparently unaffected, suggesting signs of avoidant attachment patterns (Ainsworth et al., 1978; Howe et al., 1999). It can be very easy to mistake avoidance and over-compliance for genuine 'resilience'.

8.   Research and practice show that one of the most distressing aspects of being in the care system is the experience of broken attachments, leaving children with an underlying sense of impermanence and low self-esteem (Sellick et al., 2004). Maintaining contact with people with whom they have had loving relationships has been cited by young people themselves as increasing self-worth and a sense of 'mattering' to people (Freeman, 2011). This may particularly apply to children who remain in the care system, but it also applies to adopted children, who – however much they are loved – with their history of broken attachments are also vulnerable to underlying feelings of being displaced, unloved and insignificant (see for example Triseliotis, 1983; Brodzinsky et al., 1993).

Conclusion

Our research is not offering a prescriptive solution to how moves to adoption should be carried out – and of course, all children and all moves will be different. We are also aware of the small scale of this research, and believe that much more research in this field is urgently needed. However we do believe that current procedures are out of sync with some of the fundamental principles established in attachment theory, and we would urge for a re-thinking of these procedures to bring them into closer harmony with what we know about attachment and loss. This would involve, at the very least:

- a commitment to maintaining the child's relationship with their foster carer throughout the transition and beyond, providing extra support around this if needed;
- a commitment to promoting and nurturing the foster carer/adopter relationship over the long term to facilitate the continuing involvement of the carer in the child's life;
- increasing support and training for foster carers and adopters on attachment and loss in childhood, which continues after the child has moved;
- more training across the network on recognising and responding to unspoken or latent feelings in a child or infant faced with loss or separation who appears to be 'fine';
- more training across the network in understanding the impact of organisational defences and how they can lead to blind spots when faced with pain and loss.

In the turmoil of loss and change, with new parents who are still relative strangers to them, it is not surprising that children lack the security or confidence to find ways of expressing their feelings – whether distress, chaos, anger or fear. It is our task to be emotionally attuned and responsive to the complex emotions they will be experiencing, and provide them with an environment that allows space and time for feelings of excitement and hope, but also for painful feelings of loss and confusion. If we cannot help them with this, there is a danger that they may shut down their more painful feelings and then fail to receive the comfort and reassurance they need. We strongly believe that this process of grieving and being comforted will be invaluable in helping them to develop closer and more loving relationships with their new parents; and that having their feelings understood will give them the best chance of experiencing the kind of 'continuity of existing' which, in Winnicott's words, allows people to develop an ongoing 'sense of self', and of 'feeling real'.

Editors' afterword

Much of the theory in this chapter is attachment theory, which lends itself to this topic. However, when it comes to thinking about grieving, the heart of the transition process, the authors turn to psychoanalytic theorists such as Freud, Klein and Hindle. Gianna Williams, a child psychotherapist, has written about a teenage boy in the care system who prides himself on showing no feelings of loss when he is moved from foster carers to a children's home (Williams, 2005). She points out that he *needs* these defences to protect himself over a number of different placements. We do not know if it would be practical, but it would interesting to research the move from *birth parents to foster carer*. There is a growing awareness that birth parents need support to grieve, and groups for birth parents have been set up. This is humane, but also practical, as they are less likely to rush into another pregnancy.

This chapter also attempts to address blind spots (see also Chapter 11). Behaviours that are counter-intuitive can only be understood by getting hold of more unconscious processes. In this chapter, the key point is that, in the haste to place young children with adoptive parents, the child's relationship with the foster parents is lost or minimised.

One of us worked with an adoptive mother whose child spent its first few days in an intensive care unit and then briefly with a foster carer. The transfer was quick, and in the desire to make the child theirs, the adopters had not kept up contact with the foster carer who had mothered her child during those early months. The child, now nine, suffers from physical disabilities and some learning disabilities. Over the years she had attributed the learning disabilities to the time in ICU and drug withdrawal. One day, as we were talking, she said 'I know it is organic, but there is something else. He's very bright really. But it's like he never learned the letter "a". He knows all the other letters in the alphabet but without the 'a' many words just can't make sense.' Cudmore and Boswell are interested in children who 'lose their letter a' and through their research have tried to explain the personal, professional and organisations' defences, the 'blind spots', designed to protect against the pain of loss and separation on every level.

Historically, when 'foster parents' became 'foster carers' there was a symbolic shift. It included an idea that adults looking after children out of their birth (or adoptive) families should not become too emotionally involved. This idea is still around today, when being 'professional' gets equated to being cut off from emotional states. It was rarely considered that this might have been more about protecting the adults rather than the children. At the initial introductions there is an appreciation of the importance of that early relationship with the foster carers. Yet from this research we start to see how that gets lost as both parties build defences to protect from the pain.

Foster carers can often experience burn-out. They have to drop one child in order to make space, in their home as well as their heart, for another in quick succession. Limited resources mean that they cannot get paid for the time spent in transition, and that there is no time or support for grieving. It often feels easer to drop the child from mind; to forget rather than remember.

Adopters, first appreciative of the quality of care that was provided, can come to have their own ambivalence about continued contact – a concrete reminder of the child's past, or someone who knows their child as well as they do. This can feel competitive or cruel. The desire is to 'protect' the child from memories, rather than appreciate the need for shared memories, and protect them from the pain of not having those early memories with the child themselves.

It is interesting that this research originated in an observation that 'social work colleagues seemed unclear about the reasons why moves were carried out so quickly and there was confusion about when and indeed whether it was helpful for the child to see the foster carer again'. This again suggests that without a detailed theory of human development and the development of psychological defences, social workers cannot do their jobs properly. The editors believe that understanding more about unconscious processes can enable better practice.

Acknowledgements

We would like to thank the social workers who were part of our original research team: Meena Kumari, Amanda Slattery and Ruth Wienburg; also Nicholas Midgley, Beverley Tydeman and Giles Dhabalia who all offered invaluable advice and support along the way. We are indebted to Westminster Children's Services for supporting this project over several years; and finally, our sincere thanks go out to all of the foster carers, adopters and social workers who so generously took part.

Bibliography

Ainsworth, M.D.S., Blehar, M.C., Waters, E. and Wall, S. (1978) *Patterns of Attachment: A Psychological Study of the Strange Situation*. Hillsdale, NJ: Erlbaum.

Aldgate, J. and Simmonds, J. (eds) (1988) *Direct Work with Children*. London: BAAF.

Bowlby, J. (1980) *Attachment and Loss, Vol 3: Loss, Sadness and Depression*. New York: Basic Books.

Breier, A., Kelsoe, J.R., Kirwin, P.D., Beller, S.A., Wolkowitz, O.M. and Pickar, D. (1988) Early parental loss and development of adult psychopathology. *Archives of General Psychiatry* 45(11), 987–993.

Brodzinsky, D., Schechter, M.D. and Henig, R.M. (1993) *Being Adopted: The Lifelong Search for Self.* New York: Anchor Books.

Burnell, A., Castell, K. and Cousins, G. (2009) *Planning Transitions for Children Moving to Permanent Placement: What Do You Do After You Say Hello?* London: Family Futures Practice Paper.

Dozier, M. (2007) Caregiver commitment in foster care. In Oppenheim, D. and Goldsmith, D.F. (eds) *Attachment Theory in Clinical Work with Children: Bridging the Gap between Research and Practice.* New York: Guildford Press, pp. 90–108.

Emanuel, L. (2006) The contribution of organizational dynamics to the triple deprivation of looked-after children. In: Kenrick J., Lindsey C. and Tollemache, L. (eds) *Creating New Families: Therapeutic Approaches to Fostering, Adoption and Kinship Care.* London: Tavistock Clinic, pp. 239–256.

Fahlberg, V. (1994) *A Child's Journey Through Placement.* London: BAAF.

Fratter, J. (1996), *Adoption with Contact: Implications for Theory and Practice.* London: BAAF.

Freeman, C. (2011) *Now and Then: Reflections on Relationship from Adults who Were in Care and Their Carer.* Unpublished doctoral thesis.

Freud, S. (1917) Mourning and melancholia. In *The Standard Edition of the Complete Psychological Works of Sigmund Freud, Volume XIV (1914–1916).* London: Hogarth Press.

Hindle, D. and Shulman, G. (eds) (2008) *The Emotional Experience of Adoption: A Psychoanalytic Perspective.* London: Routledge.

Howe, D., Brandon, M., Hinings, D. and Scofield, G. (1999) *Attachment Theory, Child Maltreatment and Family Support: a practice and assessment model.* London: Macmillan.

Klein, M. (1940) Mourning and its relation to manic-depressive states. *International Journal of Psychoanalysis* 21, 125–153.

Lanyado, M. (2003) The emotional tasks of moving from fostering to adoption: transitions, attachment, separation and loss. *Journal of Clinical Child Psychology and Psychiatry* 8(3). Available from http://journals.sagepub.com/doi/abs/10.1177/1359104503008003005 [accessed 6 February 2017].

Menzies Lyth, I. (1988) *Containing Anxiety in Institutions: Selected Essays.* London: Free Association Books.

Neil, E. (2009) Post-adoption contact and openness in adoptive parents' minds: consequences for children's development. *British Journal of Social Work* 39(1), 5–23.

Robertson, J. and Robertson, J. (1989) *Separation and the Very Young.* London: Free Association Books.

Romaine, M. with Turley, T. and Tuckey, N. (2007) *Preparing for Permanence.* London: BAAF.

Rutter, M. (1971) Parent-child separation: psychological effects on the children. *Journal of Child Psychology and Psychiatry* 12, 233–260.

Sellick, C., Thoburn, J. and Philpot, T. (2004) *What Works in Adoption and Foster Care?* London: Barnado's Policy and Research Unit.

Sinclair, I., Baker, C., Wilson, K. and Gibbs, I. (2005) *Foster Children: Where They Go and How They Get On.* London: Jessica Kingsley.

Schoenberg, B. *et al.* (eds.) (1970) *Loss and Grief.* Columbia: Columbia University Press.

Smith, J. (2009) *Interpretative Phenomenological Analysis: Theory, Method and Research.* London: Sage Publications.

Triseliotis, J. (1983) Identity and security in adoption and long-term fostering. *Journal of Fostering and Adoption* 15(4), 22–31.

Wakelyn, J. (2011) Therapeutic observation of an infant in foster care. *Journal of Child Psychotherapy* 37(3), 280–310.

Williams, G. (2005) Double deprivation. In Bower, M. (ed.) *Psychoanalytic Theory for Social Work Practice: Thinking Under Fire.* London: Routledge

Winnicott, C. (2004) Face to face with children (1963). In: Kanter, J. (ed.) *Face to Face with Children: The Life and Work of Clare Winnicott.* London: Karnac.

Winnicott, D. (1986) *Home Is Where We Start From: Essays by a Psychoanalyst.* New York: W. W. Norton and Company.

PART II

The value of theory for practice

7

THE USE OF SELF IN SOCIAL WORK PRACTICE

Andrew Cooper

Introduction

Therapeutic social work practice relies on us 'using ourselves' as a resource in direct work with service users. But what do we mean by the 'self' in this context, and how do we 'use' it? In this chapter I explore some psychoanalytical answers to these questions, and present a number of case studies and clinical vignettes that illustrate different aspects of the use of self.

Effective therapeutic social work is not primarily about using theory to understand other people or ourselves. Rather, it concerns a capacity for attunement to our emotional experience of ourselves in relation to others; attunement to the flow of emotional transactions between ourselves and our service users and colleagues, which are occurring constantly, whether we choose to recognise them or not. This is why the use of self is so important. Concepts like transference, countertransference, projection and splitting can seem daunting, but they describe powerful processes that will destabilise our best intentions to practise effectively if we cannot track them and work with them as they are occurring. Equally, understanding how to recognise, track and make sense of the emotional dynamics that are always alive in our work deepens our practice, improves our performance, and our effectiveness and decision making, and helps protect us from the sometimes psychologically damaging impact of the work we do. In other words it is a core professional skill, perhaps *the* most central skill we need to develop, sustain and hone.

The chapter begins with a detailed case study of one-to-one work and a series of reflective commentaries on this unfolding story. It then offers a further case study of multi-agency practice with a family where a newborn baby was deemed to be at risk, and some further reflective commentary. Finally some brief extracts from a case and how it ended are presented. Along the way a number of key concepts are introduced, and readers interested in pursuing the more theoretical aspects of the chapter can follow up the references provided. A very helpful, concise introduction to key concepts is Marion Bower's (2005) chapter. But the focus of the present chapter is on the immediacy and power of the 'lived experience' of practice encounters, making sense of these, and the meaning of 'using yourself' as a resource in the work.

A panic attack

A social worker in a voluntary sector mental health organisation began work with a socially isolated single man in his fifties. Mr A had been referred by his GP who felt concerned about him but unable to clearly 'diagnose' his problem. The GP described the man as 'difficult' and complaining. He attended the practice frequently with relatively minor medical 'complaints' – gastric symptoms, eye infections and chest pains that did not respond to routine medication and for which tests could find no obvious cause.

The worker agreed a contract of sessions with Mr A, who accepted the offer but seemed noticeably reserved and perhaps rather cynical and suspicious of whether 'it would do any good'. After three meetings the worker felt he did know more *about* Mr A, but did not feel he had *got to know him* at all. Mr A expressed much disappointment with his life. He had hoped to be married and have children, and he felt his career had never taken off. He spoke of an older brother who had made his childhood miserable with teasing and bullying that his parents had never protected him from, and of a few friends, but the worker felt that these relationships were all very 'thin'. The worker tried to be empathic with Mr A's account of his life, but these efforts to make emotional contact with him were often met with a critical response. Mr A implied that the worker had misheard him and 'got it wrong'. At the start of each session following the first meeting, Mr A would refer to something the worker had said the previous week, and again convey his dislike and disagreement. However, the worker did not completely recognise the remarks Mr A reported him having made. It was as though they had become 'twisted' in some way and it was this distorted version to which Mr A then reacted critically.

The main feeling the worker had was the sense of Mr A's isolation and loneliness, but he felt that the sessions had not led to any proper emotional contact with the sad or emotionally isolated aspect of his client. The worker found it hard to like Mr A, and began to rather dread seeing him, feeling apprehensive about receiving yet more subtle criticism and confusing communications.

Then, during the fourth session, which on the face of it developed much as the previous ones had, the worker was gradually overtaken by an anxiety that Mr A might be suicidal. He could not really account for where this feeling came from, but it gripped him increasingly as the session progressed. Not feeling he had a real alliance with Mr A, and unsure about whether the feelings and thoughts were meaningful, he said nothing. But after the session, the worker became more and more anxious and panicky. What if Mr A attempted suicide and he had done nothing? Were his case notes written up fully? Should he be alerting the GP, but if so, on what grounds? The state he found himself in did not feel like his usual professional self, which he believed to be normally quite composed. The worker realised that he could not really 'think straight' and that something unusual had taken place, which he did not understand. He sought out his supervisor. He was fortunate to have access to a supervisor who was skilled in relationship based work. What happens if you are not so fortunate is a question I take up later in the chapter.

The supervisor listened carefully and then made some suggestions. It seemed the worker had been 'invaded' by these powerful feelings and anxieties during the session with Mr A. It did not feel convincing that this was actually the worker's 'stuff', but more that he had been 'taken over' by feelings that were definitely not his. Surely there might be reason to suppose that they did have some meaningful connection to his client? He fully acknowledged the worker's sense that he did not feel he had been able to 'make contact' with Mr A at any deeper level, and that in turn Mr A seemed to feel systematically misunderstood by the worker. So was it possible that these very powerful feelings were another form of communication, and should be taken seriously? Rather than feel too panicked, the worker might think that he now *had* made some contact with Mr A, or rather that Mr A had 'got through' to him with his deeper anxieties – it just had not happened in words, or in the way the worker expected or hoped for.

The worker felt more settled, and his supervisor suggested that he needed to test out these hunches directly with Mr A at the next session. He helped the worker to think about ways to do this, at an appropriate moment in the flow of the session. So when he next met Mr A the worker found an opportunity to say 'Now I have been able to get to know you a little, I have the sense that you often feel very lonely and isolated, and very disappointed with the way things have worked out in your life. I wonder whether at times you may feel really despairing, and perhaps have thoughts of suicide?' The impact of this remark on Mr A was definite, although quite subtle. He visibly relaxed slightly, looked hard at the worker and said simply 'Yes'.

Reflecting on the process

What can we notice and learn from this account of the work with Mr A?

Engaging and creating the frame

First, it takes time to establish a working alliance with any service user, or family. Both parties are anxious and the early meetings will be full of uncertainty, as everyone works through their worries about whether they feel they can 'work with this person'. Salzberger Wittenberg's (1970) beautifully simple and direct account of the way these anxieties are active for both worker and service user is a valuable resource that unpacks the fuller meaning of a statement by the psychoanalyst Wilfred Bion:

> In every consulting room there ought to be two rather frightened people: The patient and the psychoanalyst. If not one wonders why they are bothering to find out what everyone knows.
>
> *(Bion, 1990: 5)*

Second, while these early phases of the contact are being negotiated, the worker's most important role is simply to carry on being reliably 'there'. A consistent 'frame' for the work, a regular appointment time and place helps immeasurably, as well as an absolute commitment from the worker to honour these arrangements. Failing, suddenly changing, or being late for appointments will convey that the worker's mind is not really on the client, and likely confirm worries in the service user that they are not worth the bother, that the worker cannot tolerate whatever difficulties the service user is carrying, and so on.

Recognising and engaging with the transference

Third, the phenomenon we call the 'transference' and its companion, the 'countertransference', takes time to make itself fully and clearly known. In the case of Mr A, as in every case, there are early signs and signals, and we try to take notice of these and make sense of them. The worker very quickly had an experience that Mr A is not easy to get to know and is unable to present his problems in an open and clear way so that the two of them can 'get down to work' on some issues. Perhaps then we gain some insight into why the GP made the referral – nothing the GP offered, provided or recommended seemed to work to make things better, and in the early sessions this was the social worker's experience as well. Service users who frustrate and perhaps make experienced staff feel de-skilled are often handed over to another service. The hope is often as much that another agency will relieve the first one of the strain, anxiety, frustration and guilt associated with a lack of progress, than a genuine wish that the service user might be better helped. The referral itself may be freighted with such transferential material, and our recognition of this helps us orientate to the case we are taking on.

When a transference communication does leap to the fore, it often does so from 'left field', catching us unaware and throwing us off balance. This is the nature of the 'unconscious'. If the state of mind causing anxiety for the client were better known and understood by them and hence communicable in words, it would all be much easier for us to understand and get to grips with. But painful or frightening unconscious processes are shaped and constrained by the defences the client has evolved to manage them. The worker needs to be emotionally available to receive both the defensive manifestations (often, but not always, hostile or rejecting) of the troubling mind states, as well as the communication of anxiety, panic, despair or mental conflict that underlies the defences. In Mr A's case it seems the underlying feelings are of extreme loneliness, a fear or belief that he cannot be 'reached' emotionally, or that it will be painful and humiliating if he allows this. So he rejects efforts to reach him, and seems to make the worker feel useless, hopeless and angry. The latter 'defensive' states of mind are what the worker first receives, but later he succeeds in making some tentative contact with other layers of Mr A's mind and feeling states.

Projective identification

In the case described here, the hypothesis is that the worker's 'anxiety attack' is meaningful in a special sense, if only we can discover the meaning. It is the product of a powerful form of communication we call projective identification, in which one person succeeds in exporting a state of mind more or less directly 'into' someone else who then comes to experience this state of mind as their own while simultaneously being aware that something has ambushed them internally. Casement's (1985) characterisation of projective identification as 'communication through impact' is a very helpful and accessible discussion of this process. In the case study the worker experiences a tumult of disturbing thoughts, feelings and confusion. He has the insight to suspect that something has 'got into him' or under his psychological skin. But what, and how, and can he be sure? We might notice that in the midst of this experience he says he cannot 'think straight', and be reminded of how he had noticed Mr A seeming to 'twist' the worker's communications and feed them back to him. The worker's experience is that he is not 'himself'. This captures what being subject to an experience of projective identification is like. It is more powerful, direct and perturbing to the worker than simple projection, in which one person may attribute qualities to another in a more explicit and symbolised form, although such processes occur on a subtle spectrum of intensity (Goretti, 2007).

Containment and using the 'self' to make a difference

Once the worker has explored his experiences with the supervisor, who offers a suggestion about how to use them in the next session, the question becomes one of finding the confidence to do this. Psychoanalytic work has often been critiqued on the grounds that the worker or therapist may seem to take up a position of secretly and arrogantly 'knowing the patient' better than the patient knows themselves, or of laying claim to some 'magical' type of understanding. The reality for any thoughtful practitioner is very different. We are groping in the dark much of the time, doing our best to think about the service user, and find a way to use our experiences to increase emotional contact with the deeper layers of anxiety and distress in our clients. Any interpretation of the service user's difficulties is always provisional and tentative, and most importantly must be *tested* with them in a careful and sensitive manner. If an interpretation seems to 'hit the spot', make the patient feel understood and increase genuine emotional contact, then we can be more confident we are on a helpful track.

Mr A's response does seem to have indicated that the formulation developed by worker and supervisor was accurate. However it is useful to review and notice everything that has led up to this point. The worker's emotional receptivity is a key foundation. He was able to receive Mr A's critical and suspicious communications without rejection or retaliation; he tolerated the experience of becoming invaded by anxiety in the fourth session, and then his subsequent panicky state of mind; he used his supervisor to 'think with' in an open way; and out of this process, which unfolded over several weeks, some words took shape that, when sensitively delivered, appeared to calm the service user and reach a deeper level of distress and fear within him. This process exemplifies the psychoanalytic idea of 'containment' (Bion, 1962). It is both simple and yet subtle and complex. The steps involved in the containment process are first emotional receptivity, then tolerance of the suffering and confusion that ensues, and then an effort to think and make sense of these experiences, and finally 'returning' the experiences to their originator in a new form that they find 'digestible', meaningful and helpful. We believe that this process replicates or re-enacts something of what goes on between a baby and its mother or primary caretaker in the period before the infant has the ability use words or even symbols to help make sense of its experiences, and when projective identification (see above) is the main means by which emotional distress is communicated to the mother.

Seeking help

The worker did the sensible thing, and sought help from his supervisor. His supervisor's response was thoughtful, neutral and attentive in the service of making sense of professional experience. Unfortunately the quality and availability of supervisory or consultative help evoked here is in too short supply in contemporary social work agencies. But it is a vital element in the total picture involved in the 'use of self' in practice. The fact is we cannot do this work alone, although with experience and the right training we become better able to manage complex and difficult practice encounters without seeking help all the time. A worker who can use their psychological experiences effectively will not to be ashamed or afraid of asking for help, of 'not knowing' what is going on, or of feeling incompetent and confused. As we shall see a bit later in this chapter, struggling on with experiences like the above once lodged somewhere inside us, but unprocessed, is ultimately harmful in at least two ways: we miss vital information about how to help service users with their difficulties, and we become psychologically burdened and de-skilled ourselves.

Of course, as workers in busy, hard-pressed front line services, we do have a lot of other people on our minds, and many anxieties of our own, but these matters are not the service user's problem. Even if we are lucky enough to have access to a sensitive supervisor or manager, it is unlikely that they are available 'on demand'. Living with the uncomfortable feelings and thoughts that practice encounters throw up until we can find access to a reflective supervisor or colleague is just part of the job. Colleagues can help of course, and most offices are alive with conversations about workers' recent encounters. But just 'discharging' difficult feelings and thoughts does not usually lead to better understanding of the *meaning* of it all. A better grip on what difficult practice encounters mean is the real goal, and echoing the therapeutic helping process itself, this usually needs another thinking mind with which to work.

Thus, a key message of this chapter is that relationship-based practice is not something you can practise in isolation. The power of case dynamics requires *organisational* attention, in particular the provision of reflective supervision as a standard part of agency life. As suggested, however, in practice this is often not available. So what is to be done? This is really a topic for another chapter, but one line of thought which owes something to Group Relations thinking is to say that as professionals we need to 'take our own authority' in asking our organisations for what we believe we need in order to practice well. Modern social work managers are hard pressed people, but we can expect them to listen to us in a thoughtful manner – just as our service users have the right to expect this of front line staff.

Two recent research studies that examine in minute qualitative depth the experiences of front line child protection workers show how they may become in effect 'secondarily traumatised' because of the long term impact upon them of particular cases which they found impossible to process or make sense of (Noyes, 2016; O'Sullivan, 2017). A classic text that also brings alive the experience of front line social work practice in a statutory setting is Janet Mattinson et al.'s (1979) *Mate and Stalemate*. This book was based on action research undertaken in a London social services department in the late 1970s, and while some aspects of the service context now seem dated, the processes illustrated are as recognisable as ever.

So, what is this 'self'?

The above discussion might reassure readers that when we speak about the use of self in social work, we are not referring simply to 'gut feelings' or even 'intuition', although both these notions play a part in the bigger picture of the professional self I am advancing in this chapter. The self I am interested in here is more a process than a 'thing'. It concerns our ability to scan, monitor, reflect upon, make sense of and put to work our awareness of occupying a *total field of experience* (Ogden, 1999) in what I hope to have conveyed is a sophisticated and above all thoughtful and reflective manner. This 'field' is not just subjective but inter-subjective, which means that we are attending to the continual impact of ourselves on others, and them upon us. These relationship impacts are active at the conscious, pre-conscious and unconscious levels of our own and others' experience.

Our task as workers is to know ourselves well enough, so that we can disentangle the influence of others upon ourselves, and us upon them, and thus make sense of how their anxieties, conflicts and distress are being communicated. This distinction is partly captured by the idea of distinguishing the 'personal' countertransference (what we might be projecting into our own perception of a situation) from the service user countertransference (our registration of what they might be projecting into us). Personal psychotherapy is the most helpful way a worker can evolve the deeper capacities for 'knowing themselves' that I am speaking of here. But there are other routes to deeper self-awareness, including some that reach parts of the self which individual therapy does not. Undertaking an experiential Group Relations Event in which a large body of people come together, with a staff group of facilitators, for the sole purpose of studying their own behaviour and experiences in groups and inter-group processes, are one such route. The experience of undertaking an infant or young child observation, or being a member of a 'work discussion group', are others. These experiences are not psychotherapy but especially in combination, their impact on the development of the worker may be very similar.

However, good social work and sound decision making cannot rely solely on the use of self as it is conceptualised here. We need our more cognitively oriented rational analytic faculties too in order to make sound assessments, decisions and plans. Knowledge of child development theory and research, and organisational theory are crucial, and appropriate (though not unquestioning) respect for agency procedures is vital. There is a helpful discussion of the important balance to be struck between 'intuition' and 'reasoning' in Eileen Munro's work, including her reports into the state of the child protection system (Munro, 2010).

At the sharp end

How can we use the self in pressurised, multi-disciplinary, front line service contexts, when the opportunity to create a stable frame may be compromised and urgency, risk and unexpected demands may undermine our best efforts to plan the work carefully? In a performance driven and risk-averse practice culture, can therapeutic social work really still find a foothold? The answer is definitely 'yes', but few writers have really tackled this. Heather Bailey's (2015) paper is an excellent account of how a worker can make huge advances in understanding of a complex case through thoughtful reflection and following through on an urgent, unplanned and rather crisis-laden phone call. The 'crisis' led Bailey to re-evaluate the kind of provision a traumatised child might need in order to feel contained and be able to develop.

In another paper about the Victoria Climbié report (Cooper, 2005) I focused some attention on one passage from the mass of evidence and analysis presented. It concerns the evidence given by a senior social worker, which is first quoted, followed by some commentary of my own:

> The third strategy meeting recommendation to seek some proof that the child was Kouao's, arose from a feeling she had when Kouao came into the office on 2 November that something was amiss in the interaction and bonding between Kouao and Victoria.
>
> (The Stationery Office, 2003: 179)

> [Later this worker is directly quoted:] 'Part of me, with the feelings I got from the visit with mum, it must have been still something that was niggling at me and I suggested just to be on the safe side, just to be certain, just to make sure, that she was not returned to Manning's.'
>
> (The Stationery Office, 2003: 187)

The reason these short passages spring out is that they demonstrate, in the context of the report, a rare quality of emotional aliveness to the situation facing the worker. Something troubling, and perturbing is registered and is being thought about. This speaks to what it means to have, and make use of a professional relationship in child protection work. Through an emotionally alive relationship with the family, it is possible to access something of the nature of *their relationships*. In registering a sense of disturbance, a practitioner registers signs of the potential risks, dangers and disturbances in the family relationships. Such experiences are not sufficient grounds on which to act of course, but they are necessary information which when ignored or reasoned away may be the first step on a path to tragedy.

(Cooper, 2005: 159)

Here we see an illustration of how crucially important it can be for a worker to trust her feelings, even if she can't articulate their meaning very coherently. This case eventually ended in tragedy, of course, but without doubt the social worker quoted here made the right decision at the point in time where she had the opportunity.

A baby at risk? A worker keeps her head

A social worker in a busy children's services referral and assessment team was 'collared' rather anxiously and urgently by her manager as she came into work. A referral had been made by the local hospital maternity unit who were concerned about the parental care of a newborn baby boy with Down's syndrome. The main worry seemed to be the baby's father, who was described as extremely angry, blaming the hospital staff for somehow causing his son's condition, and unable to relate to or hold the child. The baby's mother was also causing some concern. She had shown signs of bonding with her newborn, but was also distracted and had failed one opportunity to visit her baby who was still in hospital.

The manager asked the worker to make an urgent visit to the family home to meet the parents and their two-year-old daughter, and then attend a professionals meeting at the hospital. On the basis of the hospital team's experience of the 'aggressive' father, she advised strongly that the worker be accompanied on the home visit by a male social worker 'to protect her from violence'. Here, once again, we see that powerful feelings and anxieties are embedded within the referral process. The worker writes:

> However, I was concerned that an image of this family was being presented to me before I had even had any opportunity to connect with them. I was being invited to be fearful and defensive before I had even met the family, as if a state of mind that may have belonged to the hospital staff was being projected into me.
>
> I decided to make contact with the father before the arranged visit because I felt that if effective work was to take place with this family, an atmosphere of

fear and anger needed to be avoided as much as possible. When I phoned father and spoke to him, my impression was of a man who certainly was angry but also expressed a lot of vulnerability. In my countertransference I did not feel afraid of this man, but concerned for what the family including the mother and the two year old were going through in this major life changing trauma.

I think with hindsight this initial phone call and the feelings that I got from it that contrasted with the feelings I was being invited to have by the hospital professionals, was crucial in developing an effective therapeutic relationship with this family. It was as though I was able to then treat them as a family suffering as opposed to a family on the attack, and they were more able to welcome me in to the family as a potentially helpful figure.

(Erdogan, 2016)

At the meeting with the family the father remained angry and blaming of the NHS and the system. It emerged that the mother had never been offered, or maybe had not taken up, the chance of a second routine test to establish whether the foetus was healthy or not (the first test had been negative). Language difficulties may have played a role in this oversight.

After introducing myself, father asked if I knew what happened. By this it became clear that what he meant was how the hospital had let him and the family down in not being informed about the disability of the baby before birth. He said, 'You killed me, you killed my family, we are dead'.

At that point I was clearly part of 'the system' undifferentiated from the hospital staff who he felt let down by. I reflected and acknowledged his anger and said: 'You seem to be very angry, feel let down by everyone and might wonder if I will let you down too?' The latter part of my comment addressed the man's lack of trust towards me in the transference in a direct way, which may have helped him feel that at least I was not going to avoid painful and difficult feelings. The sense of unknown was very powerful and included my own feelings of facing the unknown with this family, and I used this to say something about how hard and powerful it is to be suddenly faced with such an unknown painful experience as suddenly having a disabled child.

(Erdogan, 2016)

When she meets the hospital maternity team the worker is confronted by a fresh challenge.

The number of hospital staff involved in my various meetings with them was always surprisingly high. The hospital child protection nurse who chaired the meeting outlined their concerns and there was particular emphasis on father's verbal violence to hospital staff and his lack of bonding with baby. From the outset all the hospital staff spoke with one voice. They were also concerned about mother not visiting during day time or staying at night. The idea of the baby being taken into care was put forward as the solution from the very beginning.

On reflection, it was as though hospital staff had made up their minds about what should happen, and my role would have been to implement their decision. By contrast, I fed back to the meeting my views about the home visit, agreed that father was clearly very angry but thought that such a big decision might be premature for a family who are still at early stages of coming to terms with very traumatic event. I said 'We have to give this baby and her family a chance', and that placing the baby even temporarily in care would harm the bonding relationship rather than help it.

That challenge to the overriding opinion of the meeting seemed to permit some other professionals to break away from the fixed idea that placing the baby in care was the best option, and I received some support for my suggested course of action. We ended the professionals meeting deciding that there needed to be further assessment and observation of the parents' interaction with the baby and agreed to meet the next day.

(Erdogan, 2016)

From this point on, the case begins to take its more hopeful course. The worker meets daily with the family over a period of two or three weeks, father and mother start to bond well with the baby, and everyone's anxieties about risk recede. The worker is able to engage both parents in the necessary grief work associated with their loss – loss of a much hoped-for healthy second child.

Reflecting on the process

What more can we learn from this story? Many of the same thoughts we considered in relation to the first case study apply. In effect, through astute and composed understanding of the transference forces active in the case before it has really crossed the boundary of her agency, the worker keeps her head, steadies the thinking of a complex professional system that has somewhat 'lost its head' with anxiety, and establishes a therapeutic contract with a family in great distress who are at risk because a reactive professional system has stopped 'thinking'. When she meets the father of the family, she finds a form of words that speak to his anger, his sense of being let down, and crucially locates *herself* within this transference-based interpretation – 'You seem to be very angry, feel let down by everyone and might wonder if I will let you down too?'

Because she succeeds so well in staying calm and thoughtful, it becomes easy to feel critical of the hospital team, and perhaps label them risk-averse, or over-anxious. Once the social worker has got hold of her side of matters, a more balanced view would consider that different parts of the whole professional system around the family are 'carrying' different aspects of the case dynamics. While the hospital team is acutely identified with the vulnerability and needs of the baby, the worker is in touch with the same qualities in the parents. The worker is more hopeful about change and the parents' potential, and the hospital more pessimistic. The case dynamics become split very quickly, and might have remained so had the social worker not handled these dynamics as carefully as she did. The task is to try to meet in the middle, not in a spirit of compromise, but because to make a sound assessment and decision the whole system needs to be in touch with as many dimensions of the emotional dynamics as possible.

This reflection points up how, because we are always working as a part of systems and networks, we must be capable of standing outside ourselves and seeing how we may be caught in a systemic split. Sometimes this is called occupying a 'third position'. This is not easy, because the power of the feelings of identification with one or another side of a split picture can be immense. These often reflect, but are also not reducible to, a dynamic between parents or carers in the family situation. Workers make a contribution to the strong patterns of feeling and conflict that are mobilised. Roger Bacon's (1988) paper 'Countertransference in a case conference' explores such dynamics in some depth, and Woodhouse and Pengelly's (1992) book *Anxiety and the Dynamics of Collaboration* examines how these projective and splitting processes can play out among different professions in a fixed manner, making collaboration almost impossible. Something of this is visible in the case study – the hospital team hold a conviction about the risk to the baby, but want the social worker to take on the painful and difficult task of 'taking the baby into care', thus relieving them of having to think further about the case. However, the worker succeeds in handing this projection back, and insisting quietly that they must all continue to think together, rather than rush to premature action.

There are real risks in becoming caught in dynamics like these. Feeling ourselves to be 'recruited' or pressurised into joining the 'groupthink' we will be inclined to either comply or rebel, but neither response is helpful, and risks us losing sight of vital elements of the family's situation. The skilled use of self is, in the end, about sustaining a position of independent but connected thoughtfulness.

Conclusion – and endings

The use of self in social work is central to successful practice. Over the course of a sustained piece of work, the complexity and subtlety of the processes involved will take many forms. In more conventional therapeutic work, where there is the opportunity to maintain a stable and consistent treatment frame over a long period of time, transference and counter transference dynamics can be observed and worked with more easily than in circumstances where statutory responsibilities and anxieties are mingled with the therapeutic process. Nevertheless, when a genuine therapeutic attachment forms it is vital not to lose sight of how significant you, the worker, become for the service user, and thus how important the ending of a piece of work will be for them.

A social worker who undertook a lengthy assessment of Anna, a young woman who had applied for a Special Guardianship order with respect to her niece, was able to explore the applicant's strengths and difficulties in depth. This was a process the young woman undoubtedly found very valuable. For example the worker wrote:

> When Anna was able to 'think' and 'reflect' on her feelings and actions, she became less guarded, she opened herself to new realities, new possibilities.
>
> During session six, Anna told me that she had renewed contact with her brother who she had not spoken to for the past two years, she stated 'I kind of realised that the reason he had not contact me, was maybe because I had been a bit stand offish with him, maybe he thought that I did not care, that I did not want to talk to him. Anyhow he told me he loved me at the end of his Facebook message, do you want to see it?'
>
> *(Harris, 2014)*

At the end of the assessment, the worker decides she cannot recommend Anna to be a special guardian, and clearly this affects how the process of ending the work unfolds.

> In our last two sessions, Anna appeared more guarded and less trusting, I associated this with Anna reading in my assessment my identification of her vulnerability and difficulties and her disappointment with my decision. Even though Anna was more guarded, she was able to make good use of our meetings. Mostly we explored Anna's feelings and difficulties in coming to terms with the fact that her niece was in foster care and would be adopted if Anna's appeal were not successful.
>
> I had offered to meet with Anna until the end of the court proceedings. She came to two further sessions but did not attend the subsequent ones. Somehow this felt like a natural ending. Anna was now focusing on her appeal; understandably she may have felt that communication with me may have further diminished her chances of success.
>
> *(Harris, 2014)*

At the end of any meaningful therapeutic process, the patient or service user will often start to miss, or be late for appointments. Unconsciously, perhaps, the message is 'If you can leave me, then I can do the same to you'. The worker needs to stay close to her countertransference and understand that her own feelings of disappointment or frustration at missed sessions are most likely another instance of 'communication by impact' or projection. A 'good' ending, is not necessarily a smooth or comfortable one. But as therapeutically aware social workers we are not in the business of seeking out gratitude or emotional reward of any kind, although of course it is pleasing if this is conveyed. Our task is to use ourselves reflectively, maturely and professionally.

Editors' afterword

Andrew Cooper shows that potentially life-saving insights can arise when a social worker attends to their emotional response to a client. In this case the social worker's hunch that the client was feeling suicidal was proved to be correct. One of the editors has a notebook which says 'Trust your crazy thoughts' on the front. This is something we all need to keep in mind when working with difficult or uncommunicative clients. These thoughts are often not crazy, and psychoanalysis has a word for them – *countertransference*. We would add a further element to the story of the social worker and the Down's syndrome baby: we think the hospital were feeling unacknowledged guilt and wanted to get rid of the baby, under the guise of better care. Their impermeability provoked the parents. In contrast, the social worker's willingness to be blamed calmed the parents.

Of course it is very easy to advocate being in touch with our feelings about clients, but most of us, at least initially, need support. Unfortunately the very important links between social workers are disrupted by 'hot desking', high rates of sickness and the use of agency staff. There has never been a time when psychodynamic supervision was freely available. Social workers need to fight, and maybe pay to get what they want. However there are things that can be done in any agency. Insist on regular supervision from your manager. Organise a peer-supervision group. Finally – this is something to organise for yourself – do a process recording. After your meeting with a client write down everything you can remember, including your crazy thoughts and feelings. These may give important clues about your clients. Doing this sort of exercise gets easier with practice. It is time-consuming, so probably best to confine it to your most worrying cases. At the same time, if you are mysteriously not worried by a case, this may be a worry in itself.

References

Bacon, R. (1988) Counter-transference in a case conference: resistance and rejection in work with abusing families and their children. In: Yelloly, M. *et al.* (eds) *Social Work and the Legacy of Freud*. Basingstoke: Macmillan, pp. 185–201.

Bailey, H. (2015) 'I want my social worker'. One child's struggles to find an available maternal figure: reflections from a peer supervision group. *Journal of Social Work Practice* 29 (2), 223–229.

Bion, W.R. (1962) *Learning From Experience*. London: Karnac.

Bion, W.R. (1990) *Brazilian Lectures: 1973, Sao Paulo; 1974, Rio de Janeiro/Sao Paulo*. London: Karnac.

Bower, M. (2005) Psychoanalytic theories for social work practice. In: Bower, M. (ed.) *Psychoanalytic Theory for Social Work Practice: Thinking Under Fire*. London: Routledge, pp. 3–14.

Casement, P. (1985) Forms of interactive communication. In: *On Learning from the Patient*. London: Routledge, pp. 72–101.

Cooper, A. (2005) Surface and depth in the Victoria Climbié Inquiry Report: exploring emotionally intelligent policy. In: Cooper, A. and Lousada, J. (eds) *Borderline Welfare: Feeling and Fear of Feeling in Modern Welfare*. London: Karnac, pp. 145–169.

Erdogan, E. (2016) Personal communication.

Goretti, G.R. (2007) Projective identification: a theoretical investigation of the concept starting from 'Notes on some schizoid mechanisms'. *The International Journal of Psychoanalysis* 88(2), 387–405.

Harris, L. (2014) Personal communication.

Mattinson, J., Sinclair, I., Coussell, P. and Morley, R. (1979) *Mate and Stalemate: Working with Marital Problems in a Social Services Department*. London: Basil Blackwell.

Munro, E. (2010) *The Munro Review of Child Protection. Part One: A Systems Analysis*. London: UK Government.

Noyes, C. (2016) *Live Work: Creativity on the Front Line*. Professional Doctorate thesis, University of East London and Tavistock & Portman NHS Foundation Trust.

Ogden, T.H. (1999) *Reverie and Interpretation: Sensing Something Human*. London: Karnac.

O'Sullivan, N. (2017 forthcoming) The dichotomy of 'thinking' and 'doing' in social work practice with neglected infants and toddlers. Professional Doctorate thesis, University of East London and Tavistock & Portman NHS Foundation Trust.

Salzberger Wittenberg, I. (1970) *Psychoanalytic Insight and Relationships: A Kleinian Approach*. London: Routledge.

The Stationery Office (2003) *The Victoria Climbié Inquiry Report*. London: The Stationery Office.

Woodhouse, D. and Pengelly, P. (1992) *Anxiety and the Dynamics of Collaboration*. Aberdeen: Aberdeen University Press.

8

CRISIS, WHAT CRISIS – AND WHOSE CRISIS IS IT ANYWAY?

A psychoanalytically informed account of how to keep thinking in the face of the day-to-day work of managing rising anxiety

Gill Rusbridger

In this chapter I want to talk about what triggers the need for action in working with a child, adult, or family. What is seen as needing to be managed or resolved, and in whom? Social workers are often being asked by others to step in and bring about change at a point of crisis. Something has to be done to alleviate or get rid of something that is causing anxiety or disturbance – but what is it and to whom does it belong?

I am going to illustrate this question through a case example, where the referred 'problem' that needed attention involved an 8-year-old girl whom I will call Jade. Jade's social worker asked the local CAMHS team to offer Jade some counselling, following an incident in a neighbour's flat where an alleged sexual assault on Jade by a boy of a similar age to Jade had taken place. The investigation had concluded that there were no safeguarding concerns following police checks on both families, including Jade's father, and a parenting assessment of Jade's mother, Ann. The social worker planned to close the case once the referral had been made. The alleged assault on Jade had however provoked subsequent concern in both professionals and in the family. Since then, Jade had been fearful of going out alone, and her school attendance had dropped. Her mother, Ann, was outspokenly angry and demanding that they be transferred out of their council accommodation to somewhere safe, away from the other family. Action was called for to alleviate the anxiety that had been generated.

Four meetings

The first meeting

I decided to arrange to meet initially with Jade's mother alone to find out more about what had happened and how things were now.

Ann arrived 20 minutes late for our appointment. She was a white British woman who I thought looked older than her 36 years. She was extremely anxious: sweating, trembling and talking loudly at me, almost shouting most of the time. I encountered a woman who left me feeling anxious and confused. I could barely understand what she was telling me: her speech seemed garbled and almost incoherent. I had no clear sense of what had happened to Jade. The only information that seemed to stick in my mind was that at one point she told me, in passing, that she had grown up in care and had herself been abused on numerous occasion in different settings. As a result, she did not trust professionals and glared at me in a challenging way. She was suspicious when I suggested, hesitantly, that we might need to meet again and have longer to talk.

The second meeting

I managed to arrange to see Ann again. This time, she arrived on time and seemed more available for thinking. She apologised for having 'lost it' with me last time – she felt much calmer today, partly because Jade's father had agreed to help her by collecting Jade from school each day and escorting her past their neighbour's flat. Jade's father, Dinos, was an older man of Greek descent in his forties, from whom Ann was separated, but remained friendly with – a benign but somewhat belittled figure from the description she gave me at that time. I heard that Jade was reluctant to go with him and could be aggressive and abusive towards him and clingy and tearful with her mother. I spoke about how upset everyone was and how much they might all need help to work things through. Ann seemed helped by this and agreed that we should all meet together. I suggested that I would help them to see how to co-parent Jade more effectively, and to assess Jade's emotional state, which Ann was very worried about. She left thanking me, and I felt relieved and that I was doing a good job.

The third meeting

Although I had arranged to see Ann with Jade and Dinos, Ann came to the appointment with a reluctant Jade and no father. Ann told me in a dismissive tone that Dinos had had another appointment, which she didn't believe. Jade looked doubtfully at me and wandered around my room in a wary way, as if she didn't plan to stay for long. When there were noises outside in the corridor or from the window, she started and looked anxiously at her mother for reassurance. Ann pressed her to talk to me, but this made Jade even more nervous. Eventually, when I spoke more with Ann, Jade relaxed a little and sat down and began to draw. Her picture was a stylised representation of a house with a line for the grass and a line for the sky, complete with a flower and the sun. I commented on the happy scene she had created and she smiled at me in a more connected way. I asked her some neutral questions about where she lived, were there flowers and grass, did she have friends, what did she like to play? She launched into a garbled account of a game at school with friends that I couldn't understand at all. Ann looked as though she understood everything and I felt excluded and confused. When I tried to clarify, Jade looked frightened and clammed up again, glancing at her mother and announcing that she needed the toilet. I felt I had been overly intrusive, and that I had asked too many questions, said something wrong and clumsy and had mis-understood Jade's attempt to communicate something back to me. Ann took Jade out and after some moments more back in the room it was time for them to leave. Jade wanted to take her picture with her. I suggested I keep it for a further meeting but they both looked doubtful. I said that we had started to get to know each other but that nothing felt very safe or reliable. This seemed to remind Ann about Dinos's unreliability, rather than feel reassured by me and she became rather angry again. She turned to Jade and said that Jade was being very difficult towards Dinos and wouldn't go with him: she didn't know what to do about this. Jade looked downhearted and ashamed. I felt angry with Ann for raising this dilemma when they were on the way out. I could do nothing to change their disappointment in me other than to restate that I could see that there was a lot to work out and that I hoped to see them again soon, this time with Dinos as well.

The fourth meeting

None of the more constructive work that I had hoped might take place next subsequently came about. What followed were a number of cancelled and missed appointments, with Ann gradually withdrawing and disappearing. I felt disturbed and worried, not knowing what had happened to cause the breakdown between us. Eventually I rang Ann again some weeks later. This time when she agreed to come back and see me on her own, she managed to carry this through. I did not at this stage want to include Jade and risk exposing her to more distress when I felt I couldn't predict what sort of state Ann was in.

When I saw Ann, she sounded flat and talked of Jade becoming demanding, aggressive and unmanageable. She didn't shout or appear angry during this meeting but seemed worn down and hopeless. Dinos had disappeared after she had had a go at him for being unreliable and weak in the face of Jade's own attacks on him. She had fallen out with other neighbours who were causing noise and disturbance, risking being evicted herself. She talked of thoughts of suicide or running away, leaving Jade in the care of others who might do a better job than she was able to. She then seemed to gloss over the issues and said there was nothing new about these feelings of depression – they were normal for her and I should not think otherwise or get overly alarmed. I persuaded her to agree to see her GP urgently about her low mood, and arranged that I would also contact him. However, I feared that she was not really engaged and might just be going along with this suggestion in order to brush me off. I reminded her of what she had told me about her own experiences of having been abused and said that I thought her dis-appointment might be partly due to this. She looked surprised but thoughtful. However, she then appeared to shut down and said it was something she could not talk about. I was left anxious about her capacity to look after both Jade and herself, but also wondered if I was being unduly concerned and overreacting, as Ann was implying.

Some comments

In the **first meeting** it is possible to see that the crisis in Jade's life is also a version of her mother's earlier crises being revisited. On hearing about her daughter's disclosure, Ann seemed to have been exposed to a re-experiencing of her own childhood trauma. Due to her lack of capacity to separate out these events she was not coping well and came across to me as out of control, almost mad. She was angry about what Jade had been exposed to, and also remembered her own experience, although seemingly with no real connection. To me, Ann seemed to feel left in the present with the voice of an incoherent and fragmented child self from the past. I wondered whether at some level she wanted me to feel vulnerable and helpless, left in pieces and unconfident about my capacity to provide her and Jade with space in which to think about what had happened.

In the **second meeting** I saw Ann being much more able to take a position as a thoughtful parent, able to take responsibility for her behaviour, and able to access help from both her ex-partner and myself. Although her return had been possible because of Dinos's more active role, I could see that she might also have chosen a weak or denigrated partner in him, who could allow her to appear stronger and more organised, and who would not remind her of a potent and violent male presence. She could feel some remorse about her earlier meeting with me and wanted me to know that she could be different. Perhaps my capacity to have withstood her initial incoherence and to tolerate her returning to see me, like a mother might be able to do with an upset and shaken up baby, allowed for an idea of a more benign, tolerant and understanding professional/parental figure to take hold. I felt reassured that at least a part of her seemed more together and available for Jade, and I felt more hopeful that we could work on both her own traumatic experiences and Jade's. I envisaged our being able to draw on and develop Dinos's strengthened role to act as a helpful balance to my perception of their somewhat enmeshed mother and daughter relationship. She had left expressing gratitude to me and I had been left feeling more like the helpful professional that I wanted to see myself as.

Although in the **third meeting** Ann was available for Jade and more available to me, the planned structure for this meeting was undermined when Dinos did not attend. This emphasised a mother/daughter alliance and acted to exclude Dinos as an available regulator to their dyad. Presumably this arrangement would at some level have suited Dinos too. I was also not expected to challenge this as someone who was outside the family system, and my professional authority in asking both parents to attend was undermined. Jade seemed rather hypervigilant, and I noticed a similarity with Ann's emotional state in her first meeting with me. Jade was also anxious and jumpy, and when I became too intrusive and curious she seemed to collapse, become incoherent and to project her confusion into me. Jade appeared frightened of small disturbances and unexpected noises, and even after feeling a little safer she was quickly flooded again with doubt and fear when I tried to relate to her more and understand her. She was so panicked that she seemed to need, almost concretely, to evacuate the experience from her mind and body by visiting the toilet. As a result, Ann seemed to lose confidence too and to blame me for not making the situation better, and instead seemed to imply that I had caused panic and alarm in both of them. My trying to put their experience of feeling that nothing was reliable into words made this worse rather than better. We were left angry and disappointed with each other, and, worse, Jade was left with shameful feelings located painfully inside her.

In the **fourth meeting**, Ann seemed to have withdrawn and become defeated. She could not believe in a helpful contact with me and seemed to give up on herself. This may have been a repetition of some earlier hopelessness in the face of professionals failing her. My concern led me to contact another professional, her GP. This may have seemed like an abandonment to her, rather than additional support, and confirmation of my giving up as well, and passing her on to another carer.

Although this was the end of my contact with Jade and her family at that point, Ann subsequently asked to be referred again, specifically to me, when further difficulties arose when Jade's refusal to go to school became a concern. Some of the good contact I had made with her seemed to have been remembered, held on to and not totally rejected.

Some theory

The evolving scenario described above will be familiar to many working with children and families. Where is the difficulty most acute and how should we intervene? Both Jade and Ann, it seems, are trying to recover from trauma. Who should I feel most concerned for? Is my own worry getting the better of me? Trying to think, whilst finding oneself assailed by such strong feelings and reactions, is not easy.

In order to make sense of complex, puzzling and fluctuating experiences and states of mind in my clients and in myself, and in the example here of Ann and Jade, I need to have some theoretical ideas to hand that can help me with my understanding.

First and foremost, I want to keep in mind early, primitive methods that might be being used to deal with and **defend against anxiety**. These methods of defence arise from our instinctual wish for self-preservation and survival. In a state of crisis, where anxiety is triggered by an unexpected or disturbing event, early states of mind can easily be brought into play. When anxiety is too overwhelming it becomes impossible to think, and distress and frustration have to be got rid of in fantasy and lodged in someone or somewhere else. Babies and young children have to learn how to manage physical pain such as hunger and cold, and mental distress, such as fear and anger, through using a parent or carer who initially can contain this on their behalf. A reasonably responsive parent or carer can take this on for the infant, modify it and, crucially, hand it back in a more digestible form. This will model a solid foundation that helps to build secure emotional development for a young baby or child.

In conceptualising these early mental states I find the theoretical ideas developed by the psychoanalyst Melanie Klein and her followers especially helpful. I will expand on some of these ideas below. Melanie Klein (1946) used the term **'paranoid–schizoid position'** to describe the process of managing anxiety in this binary or split way, both in infancy and, to some extent, whenever we are under extreme states of emotion. In this way, a child can retain an idea of a loving mother or carer who comforts and feeds, from one who is absent and deprives and is therefore seen as hateful figure. This is a rudimentary, basic way of trying to protect him or herself against threat by dividing good experiences from bad ones. Klein's view was that the infant evacuated bad feelings about him or herself in fantasy into others, and this process she called **splitting** and **projection**.

A related theoretical concept is that of **containment**. Historically, this derives from another of Klein's descriptions of early relationships, referred to as **projective identification,** also discussed in her 1946 paper, where one person in fantasy forcefully disowns a part of themselves and locates it in someone else. This elaboration of her idea of projection was later described by Wilfred Bion (1962) as the basis of all communication. This gave rise to the idea of **emotional containment,** most fully described by Bion in the same paper (1962). Through repeated experiences of projection and introjection of split off and then reintegrated parts, it becomes possible for the development of a more stable sense of self to take place. This process is summed up well by another psychoanalyst, Hanna Segal:

> a model, based on Melanie Klein's concept of the paranoid–schizoid position and Bion's concept of the 'mother capable of containing projective identification.' In this model, the infant's relation to his first object can be described as follows: When an infant has an intolerable anxiety, he deals with it by projecting it into the mother. The mother's response is to acknowledge the anxiety and do whatever is necessary to relieve the infant's distress. The infant's perception is that he has projected something intolerable into his object, but the object was capable of containing it and dealing with it. He can then reintroject not only his original anxiety but also an anxiety modified by having been contained. He also introjects an object capable of containing and dealing with anxiety. The containment of anxiety by an external object capable of understanding is a beginning of mental stability.
>
> *(Segal, 1975: 134–135)*

Thinking more theoretically about Ann and Jade

Ann initially appeared uncontained and unheld when we had our **first meeting**. She was full of blame towards the failings in the system that had not protected or responded to Jade, but behind this was her own sense of feeling unsafe and neglected, without the care and early containment of good parents and adults in her own childhood. She had little in the way of an internal, introjected model or template of her own to draw on when faced with a stressful situation. So instead she resorted to more primitive methods of managing anxiety where failure became projected into others, who were denigrated and made to feel as helpless as she did. This was in the face of a serious breakdown in her own internal resources, triggered by Jade's disclosure. She could not take back in and process Jade's distress because of her own reawakened distress. My own feelings of incoherence early on when I first met her, and my experience of being in the presence of someone who seemed fragmented and not in touch, were all clues about these early defensive strategies of splitting and projection. Of course, such responses can be helpful in enabling communication, as in early infancy. At times this strategy had worked well for Ann in that those feelings could be defiantly banished and exported, whilst other adults, such as myself, were left having to bear feeling like the helpless or inadequate ones whose mental stability had been threatened. However, what seemed missing for Ann was a capacity to establish a more robust and reliable internal model of containment where difficult experiences could be taken in and modified.

Social workers will often be expected to tolerate these powerful projections – from both their clients and the public. Recognising that these are extreme versions of a distorted reality – for example, that social workers are seen as completely interfering and useless, unable to spot abuse and neglect – might be of some help when trying, first, to keep hold of one's own mind; and, secondly, not to do the same in retaliation. It is tempting to resort to splitting and projection oneself by, for example, blaming completely useless parents or useless other professionals, and it is hard to resist this in the face of feeling belittled or scapegoated.

I had to reassess my aims for the work that I would be able to achieve with Ann in the light of my early meetings with her. Her highly fluctuating mental state took me by surprise. After our **second meeting** I wanted to believe that I could be a containing parent to her, and that she in turn could be a containing mother to Jade. I was caught up in my own wish to repair her and to have a good outcome for my own benefit. I had to modify this wish and see it as my own need to get rid of Ann's bad experiences and have them replaced with good ones. This is a danger in the helping professions and needs checking – we want to make things better but potentially for ourselves, supporting our own idealised and omnipotent image, rather than tolerating our clients', and our own, limitations.

Perhaps Ann was giving a strong message to me, as well as herself, when she returned for the **third appointment** together with Jade. She might have been trying to see whether I would be able to contain both of them. However, she may then have felt somewhat excluded by me, as though Jade had become a rival for my attention, making a pretty drawing for me. Like a mother with too many demands on her, I then became inadequate and had to be dismissed, leaving them intact as an idealised couple, reliant only on each other. Because of her mother's lack of capacity to feel contained, Jade also could not be held by either of us for long, and resorted to evacuating and projecting her anxiety into the toilet as the only reliable and sturdy container available to her. Jade engaged in an idealised fantasy in her picture of a perfect house with sun and flowers, with all badness disappearing into the toilet; but this split could not be maintained for long.

There was also a communication about how dangerous it might be to expect too much from me if Ann were to come regularly and become dependent on me. She might not feel able to risk being let down again after repeated experiences of this in her past. There might be too much danger of my becoming an unreliable mother who turns away and leaves her vulnerable. This may explain her withdrawal from me before eventually agreeing to a fourth meeting. During it, her depressed presentation confirmed this disillusionment, and there was no space for there being a good enough and sustaining mother in either me for her, or in herself for Jade. This may have particular resonance with the sexual aspect of the abuse they may both have experienced, where a neglectful or inattentive mother could be felt to replace one who can hold things safely.

This brings us to two other centrally important and linked concepts. Firstly, the **'depressive position'**, a term coined by Klein (1935) to denote a move away from extreme splitting between good and bad aspects of a person, and a capacity to move towards these being incorporated into an image in the mind of a whole person. This inevitably means a giving up of control, a gradual mourning and loss, and an awareness of the other's separateness – for example, that the child does not have sole possession over a mother or carer, and that a parent has a life of her or his own and is involved in other relationships that exclude him or her. Our acknowledging and accepting that we are not the centre of the universe, that we have not created ourselves and that others have a separate existence is a vital developmental step. It relates to another important concept – the **'Oedipus Complex'**. Negotiating rivalry with parents or parental figures and accepting their adult status and our smallness is key to eventually becoming mature adults ourselves. We have to have some knowledge and acceptance that we cannot cross a boundary and seduce our mother or father away from their adult couple relationship with each other. We have to manage our guilt about wanting to divide them from each other, as well as control our anger at our omnipotent wishes being held in check. As with our fluctuating capacity to be more in touch with depressive position functioning, there are many times when as adults we still wish to break boundaries and play people against each other, leave someone else out, and be the one to possess and triumph over a rival. Reaching a more integrated level of depressive functioning, and not mainly having to resort to splitting is harder if we, or our clients (such as Ann), have suffered repeated episodes of trauma or abuse in early life. The added dimension of experiences of sexual abuse, where Oedipal fantasies are matched with an actual breaking of a sexual and generational boundary, can be particularly emotionally damaging. As Trowell (2000: 99) says: 'Premature sexual experience brings about emotional chaos as well as physical damage. The maturational space needed for development is grossly disorganized in consequence.'

In the third appointment, which included Jade, Ann might have felt somewhat competitive with me: we would be rivals for being a good mother to Jade, and Jade might also be a rival for the attention I could give to Ann. I was made to feel inadequate and useless by Ann and I had to be dismissed, leaving them intact as a couple, reliant only on each other. Dinos had already become absent after a brief episode of availability. Sustained pairing between a functioning adult couple who could work together, either between Ann and Dinos, or Ann and myself, was not possible. In turn, this was unavailable to Jade as a way of modifying her own raw and immature emotional experiences. This is an example of Oedipal pairing that did not give Jade a reassuring message about the reality of her being the child in the presence of available adults, but instead promoted an idea about her remaining in an omnipotent position, merged with a mother who had her own fears about adult relationships with men as being safe and desirable.

There may have been another element in the third meeting that led to such a tense and anxious atmosphere. Dinos's decision to absent himself was a concern. The presence of a potential abuser seemed to come alive for Jade when I tried to ask questions – someone who asked about normal interests and who appeared to be friendly seemed to be felt by her quickly to become someone intrusive and who had to be got away from. Ann became infected by Jade's panic but it is not clear if this had initially been projected into Jade, or whether Jade might have revealed something more worrying about her father, which neither of them could face.

Both Ann and Jade had ongoing questions about men and masculinity. Ann had chosen a partner who perhaps needed to be very different in appearance and accent from both herself and from other men she had encountered in order for her to feel able to accept him and feel safe. Jade seemed to copy her mother's wish at times to berate him and make him (and all men) useless. Her understanding of the Greek part of herself might also have been minimised and disparaged. Jade's development as a young girl, increasingly aware of her body, and its capacity to attract was growing, but in a way that seems to have been alarming to her. It is not clear what had happened in the neighbour's flat with the boy and how curiosity about a body different to one's own had become something intrusive, frightening and disturbing.

It is important at this point to introduce one last concept, that of **transference** and its counterpart, **countertransference.** It is helpful if social workers keep in touch with what they think might be being **transferred** on to their relationship from their clients' past relationships; what they are being asked to manage and contain for their clients; and what is being stirred up in them by their clients. These feelings that are aroused in the worker are largely unconscious but through the process of supervision and self-reflection they can give important clues to the state of mind of one's clients (Heimann, 1950). I could allow myself to know that Ann made me feel deeply disturbed in my first meeting with her when she left me feeling powerfully overwhelmed, helpless and unable to think. I was also left feeling inadequate during my meeting with Jade and Ann together when I experienced being an outsider to their relationship and, lastly, when I felt some helplessness during my last meeting with Ann which I turned into action by contacting her GP. These might all be seen as examples of countertransference phenomena that were useful clues to what I was being asked and was or was not able to adequately contain.

The concept of **transference** has been described since the beginning of psychoanalysis, but the way it has been understood has changed over time. Initially it was seen by Sigmund Freud (1912) as an impediment to the work with a patient, when feelings recovered from the patient's past were transferred onto the analyst. In subsequent years, however, understanding how feelings from past relationships are transferred and re-enacted in the current relationship with a patient is seen as a crucial tool in understanding, and in bringing about change.

It may not be necessary for the social worker to convey his or her understanding of what is going on in a possible transference relationship, but it can be useful to see where these powerful affects are being aroused and played out in both clients and workers.

In the transference relationship with Ann I was both idealised and denigrated at different times. One version was of an unreliable parental figure, similar to the way that she felt about other adults, including Dinos. I also seemed momentarily at times like an idealised version of a mother that she had never had. This wish was perhaps most visible during the fourth meeting, where she seemed to have identified herself with a bad mother, and wanted Jade to be taken care of by someone who could do a better job – in the transference, me. I was also making a noise about her, like her neighbours, and in the transference causing her to feel like the denigrated and unwanted one who would be evicted by me, unless she got in first. This might have been re-enacted in the meeting with Jade, with my saying it was time to end the meeting. She became more worried and perhaps almost paranoid over time about both the perceived attacks on her and her attacks on others, including me. At the last point in our contact she could no longer hold on to any good (let alone idealised) aspect. Instead, she resorted to a negative and self-destructive solution when thinking both about putting Jade into care, where she herself had been, and about her own suicide, in order to manage an unbearable state of mind, which at that point, could not be recovered from.

Crisis – what crisis?

During a crisis, anxiety is mobilised both in many individuals and in parts of the professional network. This provokes mental instability and awakens primitive ways of dealing with it – that is to say, defensive mechanisms of splitting and projection.

Using the theoretical concepts described above helps me to try to make sense in my work with children and families and in my case example with Ann, Jade and, to a much more invisible extent, Dinos's communications. These concepts also allow me to think about and use my own strong feelings to judge what might be more unconscious aspects in relationships both in the present and from the past. In turn, I can use this theoretical framework to connect with my clients' experiences and to try to help them to see what might be going on inside themselves.

In my example, the 'crisis' for Jade was also one for Ann. Had a better relationship been established, further work with Ann would have been central in establishing a safe therapeutic place for Jade to be seen in, and where Jade's own distress could have been thought about in a more separated out way, so that Ann's experiences would have been less prone to flood into and colour what had happened to Jade. Perhaps the best way forward would have been for me to acknowledge Ann's (and my) limitations and address my understanding *with her* about her fluctuating mental state. She might have been able to recognise when she was more in touch and when something was making her more at risk of feeling out of control and overwhelmed. Could I have brought this more to her attention and been a version of a container that did not become either too demanding or too unobservant? If she could have stayed more in touch with her own emotions, she might have been able to stay more in touch with those of her daughter, and to become more tolerant of Jade's erratic emotions – especially of Jade's aggression and anxiety that caused so much reverberation and difficulty in Ann herself. I might have been able to do this in a way that did not tell Ann what to do, but would have helped her to be more in touch with her emotional self. This would have modelled a more tolerant mother/container and have mirrored depressive position thinking. It may also have left room in which to explore the strengths and limitations, in a more realistic way, of Dinos's capacity to be an involved father who was not either another abuser or a castrated and dismissed part of an adult couple.

Although I was unable to pursue this further at that time, Ann did ask to be referred back to me when further difficulties emerged with Jade, which gave some hope that I had been taken in and recovered as a potential container for them.

Summary

To summarise, I am suggesting that it is helpful, indeed essential, for a social worker to monitor her or his own reactions for intense and alarming feelings, both negative and positive. These may include anxiety, sadness, fear, anger and omnipotent pleasure at being the best helper. These are usually clues to highly split versions of reality being at play and used in an attempt to deal with anxiety. It is helpful to try to be aware of being drawn into these idealised or denigrated positions and to try to keep in mind thoughts of more depressive position functioning. These include an awareness of limitations and of being able to bear doing only well enough, not perfectly. We need to look for ways to support this mindset in both parents and children, and in ourselves. Of course, it would have been possible to have given a case example with a more positive outcome, but describing an experience of managing limited engagement and change, with the potential for revisiting what might have been held on to later, is probably closer to the reality that many front line workers have to deal with.

In order for this to be possible, social workers need access to a reliable and functioning other mind in a manager and/or a team, with whom time can be taken to think in depth on the work being carried out. This type of reflective supervision is an important part of best practice for social workers because it provides containment and space in which to explore both a client's and one's own powerful feelings. Unfortunately and sadly it is all too often seen as expendable.

In this chapter I have attempted to highlight the experience of being subjected to high levels of anxiety, and the possible consequences of this. By becoming aware of these pressures, and of the defences that can be invoked to deal with them, social workers can become more able to digest these experiences, and begin to think about them and respond to them in a more coherent, mature, 'depressive' and non-crisis state of mind.

Editors' afterword

This chapter is an important first-hand account of what it feels like to be frightened, helpless, and to feel inadequate. These are the client's feelings, but they are projected so violently into the worker that she feels they are her own experience. Powerful, intimidating clients are often referred on to more 'expert services' such as CAMHS where the whole projective process will begin again. In this case Gill Rusbridger uses theory to help her understand what is happening.

When dealing with adult clients such as Ann who have been in care, it is important to bear in mind what their early experience may have been like. Their parents have failed to protect or look after them, and they may have had contact with unhelpful or even abusive professionals. All this experience must have been going on unconsciously for Ann when she meets Gill Rusbridger, and presents as agitated and incoherent. By the second meeting she has begun to have hopes for Gill. However when Jade is introduced into the meeting Ann cannot tolerate a third person. The idealised contact with Gill immediately breaks down. Jade has probably observed this process between her mother and other people before.

Sadly the whole process of passing on is repeated. Gill tries to refer Ann to her GP when she becomes depressed – in some ways a more realistic state of mind.

References

Bion, W.R. (1962) The psycho-analytic study of thinking. *International Journal of Psychoanalysis* 43, 306–310. Reprinted as Bion, W.R. (1967) A theory of thinking. In *Second Thoughts*. London: Heinemann, pp. 110–119.

Freud, S. (1912) The dynamics of transference. *Standard Edition* 12, 97–108.

Heimann, P. (1950) On countertransference. *International Journal of Psychoanalysis* 31, 81–84.

Klein, M. (1935) A contribution to the psychogenesis of manic-depressive states. *International Journal of Psychoanalysis* 16. In (1975) *The Writings of Melanie Klein*, vol.1. London: Hogarth Press, pp. 262–289.

Klein, M. (1946 [1952]) Notes on some schizoid mechanisms, *International Journal of Psychoanalysis* 27, 99–110.

Segal, H. (1975) A psychoanalytic approach to the treatment of schizophrenia. In: Lader, M.H. (ed.) *Studies of Schizophrenia*. Ashford: Headley Brothers, Ltd.

Trowell, J. (2000) Assessing sexually abused children. In: Rustin, M. and Quagliata, E. (eds) *Assessment in Child Psychotherapy*. London: Duckworth, pp. 95–107.

9

EXPLORING RACIST STATES OF MIND

Narendra Keval

This chapter explores ways in which racist states of mind serve particular kinds of psychic and socio-political functions that can be fathomed by exploring some of the unconscious phantasies which lie beneath the surface of some of the narratives in racist thinking and feeling. I suggest that these phantasies are evident in both our current social/political climate and experiences in the consulting room with some of our patients when they are temporarily under the grip of this way of thinking and feeling. Observations of these narratives can provide us with an understanding about the quality of thinking or mental space that is being inhabited by the individual, group or society at any given moment.

During the general atmosphere leading up to and following the outcome of the recent British referendum, it was difficult not to be struck by the provocative use of immigration issues that started fuelling the racist imagination in our national psyche. There were echoes of Enoch Powell's 'Rivers of Blood' speech almost 50 years ago (Powell, 1968), in which he portrayed the immigrant as an unwelcome stranger who caused psychic and social mayhem to an idealised English landscape and social order. The crude racist graffiti on the walls of Black and Asian neighbourhoods in the 1970s found new ground in the aftermath of 'Brexit' as we witnessed familiar etchings of hatred towards other communities. This was most tragically witnessed in the recent murder of a Polish man in Essex by a gang of white men who attacked him once they heard him having a conversation on his mobile phone in his mother tongue.

Since the Brexit vote there has been a staggering increase in race hate crimes in Britain. It also emboldened over 100 MEPs that sit in the European Parliament on the far right and nationalist spectrum to use the cacophony of crises from mass migration and terrorism for political capital that some have called 'fortress Europe'. Further afield, we are witnessing turmoil in American politics since the incendiary comments and actions of President Trump. He advocates for a policy of what he refers to as 'extreme vetting' and a 'total and complete shutdown of Muslims entering the United States until our country's representatives can figure out what the hell is going on. We have no choice ... we have no choice'. His solution to manage difficult issues on immigration in relation to Mexico is to build 'an impenetrable, physical, tall, powerful, beautiful southern border wall'. His racist stereotyping depicts Mexicans as drug smugglers, murderers and rapists.

Similarly, a recent newspaper article reported an inflight magazine on a Chinese airline that gave passengers visiting London, the following precautions: 'London is generally a safe place to travel, however precautions are needed when entering areas mainly populated by Indians, Pakistanis and black people. We advise tourists not to go out alone at night, and females always to be accompanied by another person' (Diebelius et al., 2016).

The abundance of spatial metaphors or imagery in political discourse that portrays building walls, fortresses, borders or fences in tumultuous times is no accident. In the face of anxieties and fears, the racist imagination seeks out idealised spaces in the mind that offer tempting retreats in which loyalty towards an imagined sense of community, tribal group, belief system or an abstraction takes precedence over the capacity for reason and empathy. These idealised spaces may picture a certain time, place and customs, free of unwelcome intrusions and frustration. The past is perceived in a nostalgic gaze that has become stuck in the belief that it was somehow better, more peaceful and calmer when there was no mixing of cultures and no need to acknowledge 'other people'. However, these intricate and elaborate defences are also designed to lay claim to an absolute version of truth that misrepresents reality.

I suggest that narratives of race hate have unconscious recurring themes that are ignited through inflammatory rhetoric and imagery, driving some of the murderousness of racism that we often witness in our society. What is striking in listening to these moral panics of recent times is that their arrogant, bullying and hysterical quality can easily provoke a wish to shut down our own capacity to think and overlook the sense of bewilderment and loss that is being alluded to in the longing for 'what once was and is no longer' – a universal theme.

One report described the cathedral city of Peterborough being under siege, with migration held to be responsible for putting pressure on public services and local resentment about the *changing character* of the ancient English settlement. In one popular street, a traditional English baker's shop finally closed after 136 years. The blame is placed firmly at the door of the new Polish delicatessen two doors down. One resident commented, 'three generations that ran this shop for over 100 years – it's gone too far – country's gone too far, this country is never going to be the same again. We can only hope that we can put a stop to it.' One Sheffield resident commented 'we've lost the steel works, coal, everything is gone, everything is going', while another commented with absolute certainty that foreigners were taking all the jobs.

In racism, social grievances (e.g. anti-establishment feeling, alienation, marginalisation, unemployment, loss of local industry and community) become the battlegrounds, but what is at stake is the sense of self. One report in the aftermath of the Brexit result showed a woman raising her fists in triumph saying 'Just glad we are going to be out – this is our England, our England' while another showed an elderly man sobbing, looking grief stricken, saying 'I have got my country back, what I've got I want to keep', believing that a vital experience to his sense of self and identity was now recovered.

It seems that the binary choice of being 'in' and 'out' of the EU gave licence for some to impose a malignant form of othering that confirmed a compelling regressive phantasy of a pure and uncontaminated Britain that could be recovered by driving so-called foreigners out. The in or out thinking in the referendum provided ample, fertile ground for the concrete thinking, splitting, evacuation and a claim to an absolute knowing that is so characteristic of racism. Getting one's country back literally meant for some to have licence to eject and evacuate others out of it.

Racist populist movements depict immigrants, refugees, asylum seekers and so on as enemies who threaten an imagined sense of community, values and 'way of life'. While these phantasies that dehumanise others in terms such as diseases, insects or vermin are felt to threaten and destroy the national body politic, what is also being alluded to in this phantasy of others as parasites is that their needs are going to invade and rob the body of the nation manifest in the paranoid anxiety such as all jobs and NHS resources being taken by foreigners.

This conveys racism's preoccupation that concretely equates the body of the ethnic other with psyche and nationhood (Reicher and Hopkins, 2001) – an equation that is clearly evident on the international stage, where geographical spaces and boundaries arouse such primitive passions (Said, 2003). In the current climate projective processes have opportunistically seized to mine the divisions of 'us' and 'them' with ease. No wonder building walls has become an obsession, allowing fundamental anxieties to do with the attacks on one's body to be exploited for political purposes to expunge 'foreign bodies', pollutants or difference (Auestad, 2016) to the other side of the wall. It is interesting that in Calais, the migrant camps where people live in squalor are called 'the jungle'.

There are many historical and contemporary examples of how racist phantasies can be exploited to create a climate of anxiety and fear because of their capacity for anxieties to be experienced viscerally like an aversion or a contamination which has to be got rid of concretely and therefore cleansed from the psyche. However, these phantasies of cleansing need to be understood in the context of a wider narrative of an imaginary love lost, feelings of bewilderment and a sense of betrayal that drives a grievance and a wish for revenge, factors that are perhaps less well explored in the motivations behind the murderousness of racism.

Gadd's sociological analyses (2010) touch on this issue when he suggests that racist hatred is a function of a complex melding of hidden injuries and hurts arising from traumatic ruptures of relationships in an individual's past with those of class-based injustices (e.g. unemployment through industrial decline leading to loss of community/income/pride/potency), resulting in a profound sense of loss.

Rejections, shame and humiliations in one domain of experience both reinforce and are reinforced by those in another. What is being suggested is that these multi-layered losses can culminate in grievances and hatreds that coalesce and find expression in a predatory, socially sanctioned and opportunistic structure in racism, which serves to bind all the emotional turmoil that is locked into melancholic responses. This formulation and others that situate racist hatred within the turmoil of socio-cultural melancholia (Gilroy, 2006) point to, but do not sufficiently explore, layers of losses which require closer scrutiny. Freud speaks to these other scenes in his classic work 'Mourning and Melancholia' (1917):

> Mourning is regularly the reaction to the loss of a loved person, or to the loss of some abstraction which has taken the place of one, such as one's country, liberty, an ideal and so on. (p. 243)
>
> In analyses it often becomes evident that first one and then another memory is activated, and that the laments which always sound the same and are wearisome in their monotony nevertheless take their rise each time in some different unconscious source. (p. 256)

Some of these deeper sources of laments in racism are what I understand to be part of the complex and potentially toxic melding of narcissistic injuries derived from both the personal and political realms of experience. The arrival or presence of the stranger or foreigner is not only felt to be a symbolic loss representing a loved person such as community, country or nationhood that was inflicted, it is also imbued with the central feeling of being psychically robbed or depleted as a result. The notion that one has got one's country back implies it was a phantasy object that was stolen, to which there was an entitlement. This grievance is further fuelled by an outrage that a couple represented by notions of a nation state, authority or establishment allowed this to happen in the first place. In this sense a perceived influx of strangers that were allowed to contaminate an idealised relationship is felt to be a betrayal for which revenge is sought. In this way the shadow of the object of grievance is projected on to the stranger.

I suggest that racist events, wherever we may encounter them, have a narrative that contain core themes which I refer to as a 'racist scene' (Keval, 2016) in which phantasies and feelings that belong to another unconscious scene (Cohen, 1993: 12) involve a toxic grievance whose structure contains: elements of bewilderment (e.g. Donald Trump's comments 'what the hell is going on?'); symbolic loss ('we have got our country back'); a sense of powerlessness ('we have no choice'); a sense of betrayal; and feelings of shame and humiliation. Notice that the official logo of Trump's presidential campaign was 'Make America great again', and his statement 'It's going to be America first, America first, America, America, America first'.

Phantasies of race in the clinical situation

Phantasies and feelings that belong to this other scene are more accessible in the clinical situation where they can be tracked and followed more closely. I suggest that preoccupations to do with difference in the form of ethnicity, race or racism and their lived experience are always present in subtle ways in the privacy of our daily thoughts and feelings, imagination and dreams. Our clinical encounters are no exception but they need close and sensitive scrutiny to capture the nuances of what is being grappled with and communicated. These deep structures of thought and feeling are universally present in contemporary culture as well as the consulting room, where they may come to constitute the passions of the transference.

Take the example of racist graffiti, seen in many urban neighbourhoods of the 1970s, which is now seeing a resurgence. Slogans that demand 'Poles go home' and 'you dirty fucking Pakis' begs the question what these crude etchings of hate are trying to communicate? Why should a couple engaged in sexual intercourse evoke such upset and outrage in the racist that they have to be ostensibly evacuated and sent home packing? Who or what does the notion of 'home' represent that is perceived to have been violated? What is the meaning of this sense of outrage in the mind?

Clinically, we are often preoccupied with the benign and malignant functions of phantasies used by the patient at different moments, often weaving in and out as they do, interacting in subtle and myriad of ways with internal and external reality. We listen for how the ambience and particular objects and features of early life use both the current setting and features of the therapist/analyst to give particular shape and form to the transference relationship. Their reference in the patient's material often signal the first signs of a deepening of the therapeutic relationship and can often act as a catalyst for exploring meaningful issues for them. I also see the use of these phantasies as telling me something about the way internal objects are being allowed to relate to each other in a lively, pleasurable or destructive way and the patient's relationship to this internal configuration. The quality of these relationships are crucial in the way they determine the capacity for thinking. Since thinking necessitates making links, a psychic intercourse, it also forms the prototype for the development of creativity as symbolised by how the parental couple are linked together in the mind (Bion, 1962; Meltzer, 1973). A capacity to link thoughts, to think and create meaning, is therefore shaped by the way the parents in the Oedipal situation are perceived and used, determining the shape of the mental space.

In this way a link has been made between the developmental tasks in the Oedipal situation and the way mental space is structured, affecting the capacity to comprehend and relate to reality. The development of curiosity and concern towards the other requires the recognition of the other as a fellow human being separate from oneself, a recognition that comes out of a particular state of mind termed the depressive position (Klein, 1946). In contrast, the paranoid-schizoid mode of functioning mobilises splitting and projection to obstruct that recognition.

Britton (1989) refers to this development in mental life as the creation of a 'triangular space', which introduces new challenges that provoke anxiety in the child's mind. If the anxieties of feeling excluded from the parental relations are manageable it introduces different possibilities, that of being an observer of the parents' relationship and allowing oneself to be observed in relation to another. This is dependent on the individual's capacity to play with different configurations of links between objects in the mind, which include the realisation of both the anatomical/ sexual as well as generational differences that are present in the triangular situation between children and parents.

I suggest that curiosity about these links and what they give rise to determines whether mental space expands to accommodate knowledge about these 'facts of life' or contracts if the anxiety is too intolerable. Changes from two-dimensional to three-dimensional thinking that reflects psychic complexity and diversity will depend on the type of anxieties dominating the individual, group or organisation at any given moment. Central to these discoveries is a capacity to bear loss and mourning as part of the recognition of one's position in the larger scheme of things that psychic complexity brings forth. It is a lifelong struggle to learn and comprehend the complexity of this ordinary human reality, a development that is thought to bring about a different conception of mental space, and quality and depth to thinking and feeling.

Consistent with the idea of benign and malignant functions of phantasies, I find it helpful clinically to make a distinction between the use of *racial* and *racist* phantasies whose functions are different. Where the latter can express a wish to evacuate, control or oppress the other, the former can reflect a wish to engage and explore the self through the other, fostering curiosity, concern and learning. I also view the trajectories of these phantasies determining to what extent the couple in the mind can be allowed to come together to engage in a productive relationship where two contrasting ideas (gendered difference) can accommodate and interact with each other without becoming violated by fusion or splitting. This would be the emotional/ psychic equivalent of sexual intercourse, in which different ideas can come together within the mind in the service of reflective and productive thinking or creativity and the capacity to manage contradiction and ambiguity (Feldman, 1989).

Clinical vignette 1

Mr A, a white male patient, spoke in a haughty manner about his fondness of living in colonial Africa and his exposure to the local black 'natives' in his neighbourhood. This was tinged with a sense of bewilderment and a facial expression of disgust about the kind of food they ate and his perception of their behaviour as dirty and unruly, which he found abhorrent. This material emerged following previous sessions in which he was grappling with whether he needed to continue his sessions or just 'pull his socks up and get on with it'. He thought asking for help was pathetic, a sign of sheer weakness which his military family would scoff at if they ever found out he was getting help.

His next comment was about his black neighbour in an apartment complex whom he was convinced had made the carpet in the foyer dirty, without any evidence for his accusation except that, being from Africa, this was probably to be expected, and all part of her normal behaviour. All this was spoken in an eminently reasonable tone, carrying with it a sign of his tolerance for other cultures, which barely hid his contempt. He then went on to tell me about how fascinated he had become with using foreign recipes in his cooking and that he found himself experimenting with these and getting too carried away with it which made him want to reign himself in. I noted how he felt his mind had been messed up by his 'native therapist' but that something productive was also happening that was making him both excited and alarmed.

His gradual discovery of my significance in his psychic life, specifically of his hunger and dependency on me was now creating a problem for his racist phantasies as part of his defensive organisation of superiority. However, this hostility to me was struggling to give some leeway towards a capacity to both accommodate and *use* me in his curiosity and willingness to experiment and enjoy his food. However, he also faced an internal dilemma that is captured in his wish to 'reign himself in' as the pleasures of feeding himself conflicted with a loyalty to his racism that gave him a feeling of superiority but kept him emotionally starved.

The following case material describes my experience of working clinically in more detail, with a patient struggling to manage feelings of separation, loss and the pain of mourning by, first, expressions of bewilderment and a narcissistic injury that led to a retreat into her racist thinking and feeling which offered her a temporary refuge from which to attack me to obtain temporary relief. This was at the cost of obstructing her capacity to become curious, concerned and productive in her life. Some of her reactions to the 'noise of diversity' and attempts to attack and spoil through revenge has resonance with reactions to diversity and difference on the wider social canvas of society. They touch on some of the core themes in the narratives of racism which I have termed the 'racist scene' as a variant of the primal scene, saturating it with complex layers of meaning. These manifest in attacks on the capacity for linking, thinking and the creation of meaning embodied within a productive coupling.

Clinical vignette 2

Ms B, a white female woman, on entering my consulting room looked at my carpet and commented 'a most unwelcoming colour' and said she preferred lighter colours (Keval, 2005). I recall how I was struck by this unexpected comment about my presence in this opening gambit of our first meeting which I later came to understand as a central feature in the way she managed herself – to evacuate rather than engage with her feelings about all aspects of her life.

The clinical material will focus on the session following a summer break when she returned with some thoughts that I had been enjoying the weather with my family and friends in the garden which had recently been renovated. She disliked that the green grass had been replaced with wooden decking. The tone of this conveyed some outrage that she was excluded from not only this change that had taken place but also the imagined enjoyment in the garden. She then said that she had a thought, which some of her white friends usually expressed, that Asians did not want to take the time and trouble to cultivate nice gardens, opting instead for easy, bland and unimaginative solutions. She said she was quite aware that it was a ridiculous thought and then spoke about her fondness for the green countryside. An early memory came to her mind, of travelling alone to her aunt's house in the summer break and watching the uninterrupted green countryside which she loved to see rush past her in the fast train but the trip was resented because she did not want to be separated from her parents.

During my break, she was unable to do any writing for her research in the library because she felt intimidated by the prospect of asking for help from the library staff and looking at people who seemed to be working hard. She found it too difficult to think about 'labouring' over her work and decided to leave the library feeling disgruntled. At one point in the break she went to London's East End for shopping and felt frustrated, resenting the unfamiliar languages and different types of foods she encountered in the shops, invaded as she put it by 'all this foreign stuff'. Although she fled from this shopping trip when it became intolerable for her she was taken by surprise by a feeling of how much she liked the way the Asian grocers talked affectionately with the old ladies. She conveyed something important about this moment in which she paused and started to 'look' in a different way accompanied by a fleeting experience of a good feeling inside her.

Ms B's struggle to cope with her feelings of loss and exclusion triggered by our separation touched and opened up many wounds in her experience that included a nostalgic gaze over her somewhat idealised past which she used as an antidote to the many traumatic experiences of her early life. This was connected in the way she oscillated between evacuation and metabolising the meaning of her relationship with me, expressed in the reactions she had to the library and to the ethnic or racial differences she faced on her shopping trip. Witnessing others engaged in productive work in the library and drawing help from staff to 'labour' over ideas for her research meant having to tolerate feeling small like a hungry infant with needs and allowing this feeding relationship to flourish in her mind as represented by a labour of thoughts and feelings.

Similarly, she was unconsciously outraged that I should have the audacity to change the garden and cultivate my interests and preoccupations that did not include her. The pain from her feelings of loss and narcissistic injury of being excluded is expressed in the conflict between the old and new/same and different. Here the wish to cling to the old and familiar was also a wish to have things back to the way they were before my summer break, reflecting a phantasy of her therapeutic 'home' that had been invaded by the unwelcome guests, puncturing what she imagined to be a relationship where only she and I existed, that excluded all else, not unlike her idealisation of the uninterrupted green pastures of the countryside. When she saw my garden on her return from the break, she felt bewildered and angry with the sudden recognition that the new garden triggered, namely that I had a separate life, independent of her. This particular version of the parental intercourse and 'noise' is reacted to by becoming superior and turning it into a 'bland unimaginative' experience to reduce the psychic noise in her mind that infuriated and injured her. She then launched an attack on her Asian therapist/ people in the East End who exercised an independence of mind and stepped out of line in choosing to speak and enjoy their language in their mother tongue ('foreign stuff') that made her small, helpless and excluded.

When overcome by her feelings of bewilderment in her encounter with the 'noise' of diversity and differences on her shopping trip, she retreated once again but this time with a warm feeling that caught her by surprise with a curious glance at the affectionate exchanges between the grocers and their customers. This echoed some of her experiences of working together with me that she valued and which survived the ravages of her racist thinking and feeling. A new and different thought and possibilities of being and looking both into herself and around her could be allowed into her mind. Instead of clinging to her grudge it would require her to take the time and trouble to recognise the value of our work and the liveliness and potency of others she witnessed on her shopping trip so that she could use us as objects to cultivate and use her own mind instead of spoiling and attacking others.

Racism in the mind and society

Ms B's initial reaction to my ethnicity was to evacuate the idea of my ethnicity/ skin colour that she could not tolerate in her mind just as she felt outraged and *escaped the scene* where 'foreign stuff' was taking place, the noise of different people and languages that in her unconscious phantasy represented the noise of a parental couple together which she found bewildering and from which she felt excluded. Similarly, her initial reactions to first meeting me in the consulting room was to evacuate from her mind the 'unwelcome colour' of my skin. Her preoccupations in the garden during the break was to attack it by turning it into a bland unimaginative 'intercourse' taking place, stripping it of any real feeling, meaning or potency. I had in her mind stepped out of line and should have *known my place*. This was not unlike her difficulty in the library of witnessing others 'labouring' over ideas which she found unbearable only to leave feeling disgruntled.

This intolerance of others' preoccupations which includes their capacity to engage in productive thinking or work echoes Britton's (1989) description of a patient who was unable to tolerate his capacity to think as an analyst; his patient shouted at him 'stop that fucking thinking'. His patient experienced and symbolically equated his analyst's thinking to an act of sexual intercourse that could not be tolerated. This resonates with the outrage expressed by the racist graffiti 'you dirty fucking Paki' that expresses a certain discovery and recognition of a couple that is felt to be forced upon the perpetrator's mind.

Some of the reactions of this patient have a certain resonance in how racist states of mind emerge in society. This patient's feelings of bewilderment were accompanied by a cocktail of feelings that included a feeling of being robbed of her therapeutic home as she left it before the break that resulted in a puncture of her narcissistic phantasy, resulting in an injury. This prompted an attack on my potency and of others, turning an imagined vibrant sexual, social and intellectual intercourse into one devoid of any real meaning. The attack on the potency of others being productive throws light on how racism organises itself both internally and in the external world, by keeping its needed objects denigrated and straitjacketed into prescribed roles so that the racist dictum is kept in force: 'Know your place' and do not step out of line.

Thuggery, both overt and covert, is always present to one degree or another in racism and can even become enacted by the very institutions that support reason and humanity. I was struck by this in the previous coalition government's strategy on illegal immigration that took the form of vans being driven around London boroughs with the slogan 'Go back home, or face arrest'. The perception and treatment of vulnerable asylum seekers as 'prisoners', or placing refugees in towns and cities of Britain without thinking through the extent to which it might fuel acrimony and racism in host communities, shows a reckless lack of foresight and compassion.

The new wall built in Calais to manage the migrant situation raises questions regarding whether it is intended to keep racist projections in place or a genuine humanitarian attempt to contain the situation. The former will ensure that vulnerable people are kept at a distance in squalid conditions, keeping them in permanent dependency and powerlessness through starving them of the most basic care. Keeping them out of sight and out of mind behind the walls bolsters the delusion that it is the migrants themselves who are responsible for their deprived conditions and squalor and do not deserve anything better. It ensures that those on the receiving end 'know their place' – denying them their identity. Any sign of protest at being dehumanised is seen as further evidence taken to justify quarantining and cordoning them off from the rest of society. The sense of entrapment in this Kafkaesque world is well known to those on the receiving end of racist hatred in which any reasonable plea for fairness made is used as evidence by the 'prosecution' that starts from a position of assumed guilt, and from there it is an uphill if not impossible struggle to establish the truth of the matter.

Concrete and psychic walls also ensure that what is kept out of sight and out of mind is a sense of responsibility and guilt for the damage wreaked towards others on the other side of the wall, not unlike my patient who could not bear to look and wanted to escape the scene of diversity. However, if grief and mourning are allowed to proceed then a new possibility arises such as a momentary discovery of warm humane feelings that enabled her to give a curious glance and perhaps recognise the value in accommodating others and recognise a common humanity.

While I have focused on racist states of mind that have emerged in our society more forcefully in recent times in the light of tumultuous events, it is important to emphasise that these 'mind states' affect all organisations to one degree or another, across our society including ones that represent our own professional practices. Professional spaces and bodies of knowledge can become too comfortable or idealised with their own perimeter walls that allow an escape from the noise of diversity and keep others deemed too different to be kept out so they know their place in the most subtle of ways.

Conclusion

Identity is a complex tapestry. As we move fluidly in our psychic identifications and geographically from one place to another so we are inextricably linked and connected. This offends the sensibilities of the racist imagination, which strives to create myths of purity that only exist in our wishful thinking for absolute certainties.

These myths are entrenched beliefs that strongly resist any mixture with the new and different, their principal aim being to obliterate linking, meaning and even life itself. Intertwined with the vicissitudes of social life, their predatory and opportunistic nature also make these beliefs extremely resistant to change. The post-Brexit triumph which for some laid a claim to recovering an imagined Britain, unblemished by foreigners, appeared to be a code word for an intolerance of not only the relative tensions, conflicts and uncertainties but also the potential pleasures that an engagement with the diversity of others can bring.

I have suggested that idealised spaces in the mind echo another unconscious scene which is saturated with complex layers of meanings. These involve a toxic melding of narcissistic injuries and grievances rooted in the feeling of being robbed and betrayed by the first forcible eviction and transition from the primordial home, into the symbolic world of language and cultural space of another. Instead of mourning these multi-layered losses, grievance and a wish for revenge takes precedence in which thwarting, robbing or expunging ethnic others becomes an endless pursuit to recover what is lost to re-create an imagined utopia. But it is a mythical structure – there is nothing to retreat to. In trying to make life apparently manageable racist hatred strangles all life.

Editors' afterword

As social workers reading a chapter on racism, it is possible to take pride for a moment in remembering that the social work discipline has been at the forefront of grappling with Racism and Institutional Racism since the early 1980s – far longer than most other professions. At the same time, social work distanced itself from psychoanalysis having an idea that psychoanalytic theory itself was racist. The curriculum of most social work courses as long as 30 years ago focused on what was then termed Anti-Discriminatory Practice (ADP). As a profession we were advocating on behalf of clients facing racism in criminal justice, mental health or social care institutions as well as championing change in political and cultural arenas. Moreover, we were soul searching in our own profession. Practice debates ensued about transracial placements, whether we were racist or culturally biased in our child protection practices, and about how to challenge the over-representation of black men in psychiatric units and prisons. ADP included the idea 'empowerment', and we saw our role as empowering our clients and the communities we worked in. The problem with those social and political theories, while central to the social work role and tasks, and a foundation for our ethics and values, was that they did not help us to figure out what to do in face to face encounters with our clients.

Keval is demonstrating to us that psychoanalytic theory, far from being devoid of ideas about race, can show us how it is useful in understanding the complex nature of racism both in the external and internal word. He invites us to notice how racism resides in the unconscious and provides us with examples of how it manifests in global political contexts as well as how it manifests itself in individual professional relationships in the transference.

References

Auestad, L. (2016) The social unconscious and the herd. *New Associations* 20, 1–2.

Bion, W.R. (1962) A theory of thinking. *International Journal of Psycho-analysis* 43, 306–310. Reprinted in: Spillius, E. (ed.) (1988) *Melanie Klein Today: Developments in Theory and Practice, Volume 1, Mainly Theory*. London: Routledge, pp. 178–186.

Britton, R. (1989) The missing link: parental sexuality in the Oedipus complex. In: Steiner, J. (ed.) *The Oedipus Complex Today*. London: Karnac, pp. 83–102.

Cohen, P. (1993). *Home Rules: Some Reflections on Race and Nationalism in Everyday Life*. London: The New Ethnicities Unit. University of East London.

Diebelius, G., Davis, B. and Newling, D. (2016) Chinese airline magazine in racism storm over article warning tourists to avoid parts of London 'populated by Indians, Pakistanis and Black people'. Available from: www.standard.co.uk [accessed 6 February 2017].

Feldman, M. (1989) The Oedipus complex: manifestations in the inner world and the therapeutic situation. In Steiner, J. (ed.) *The Oedipus Complex Today*. London: Karnac, pp. 103–128.

Freud, S. (1917) Mourning and melancholia. *Standard Edition* 14, 243–258. London: Hogarth Press.

Gadd, D. (2010) Racial hatred and unmourned loss. *Sociological Research Online* 15(3), 1–20.

Gilroy, P. (2006) *Postcolonial Melancholia*. New York: Columbia University Press.

Keval, N. (2005) Racist states of mind. In: Bower, M. (ed.) *Psychoanalytic Theory for Social Work Practice: Thinking Under Fire*. London: Routledge, pp. 30–43.

Keval, N. (2016) *Racist States of Mind: Understanding the Perversion of Curiosity and Concern*. London: Karnac.

Klein, M. (1946) Notes on some schizoid mechanisms. *International Journal of Psycho-Analysis* 27, 99–110.

Meltzer, D. (1973) *Sexual States of Mind*. Perthshire: Clunie.

Powell, E. (1968) Rivers of Blood, speech by Enoch Powell MP at a Conservative Association meeting in Birmingham, UK, 20 April 1968. Available from: www.telegraph.co.uk/comment/3643823/Enoch-Powells-Rivers-of blood-speech.html [accessed 6 February 2017].

Reicher, S. and Hopkins, N. (2001) *Self and Nation*. London: Sage Publications.

Said, E.W. (2003) *Freud and the Non-European*. London: Verso, in Association with the Freud Museum.

10

NO SHIT!

A psycho-educational group for foster carers

Robin Solomon

Research demonstrates that placement stability is highly correlated to better emotional and cognitive outcomes for looked after children (Munro and Hardy, 2006; Rock et al., 2015; Bazalgette et al., 2015; Sinclair et al., 2007). Yet placement breakdowns are all too common, and for each child a placement breakdown can often predicate further ones. When placements break down, there is a desire to allocate blame, and 'professional breakdown meetings' rigidify this process. The 'inadequacy' of carers or the extreme behaviours of the young people are often blamed. Yet it might be more helpful to think about placement breakdown as a repetition of the original experience the child has of a breakdown of a family. Every child who comes into care is there because some aspects of its birth family relationships have irretrievably broken down.

Repetition compulsion is a psychological phenomenon in which a person repeats a traumatic event or its circumstances over and over again. This includes re-enacting the event or putting oneself in situations that have a high probability of the event occurring again (Freud, 1920). In this case the young person unconsciously recreates the relationships that led to the original breakdown, and the carers get unconsciously pulled into assuming a familiar role in those repetitions.

Although a common response to a placement breakdown is an attempt to 'fix' the child by sending them for therapy, this is often unsuccessful. Since these are children for whom engaging in a relationship *is* the problem, an idea that they will engage in a therapeutic relationship is often premature. Therefore, it is sometimes more realistic to target work to maintain placement stability rather than 'change the child'. It is perhaps tautological to say the longer the child can be maintained in a successful foster care setting, the more likely that other changes may be possible. Therefore supporting foster carers and helping them to understand the children in their care could be seen to be both a more effective use of resources as well as a preferred therapeutic intervention. So what would that targeted work look like, and why has it been so difficult to provide? Perhaps because what is true for good parenting is also true of good foster parenting – to be containing, one has also to feel contained.

Establishing a model

As part of a specialist Looked-After Children CAMHS service commissioned by a local authority, I was involved in setting up and facilitating groups for foster carers with the aim of preventing placement breakdown through providing specialist training and support to the foster carers. All of the borough's foster carers already had access to a comprehensive training programme where they were required to sign up for a requisite number of training days on various topics. They also were required to attend a monthly 'support group'. Yet there was a strong feeling throughout the department that the trainings were not impacting on the quality of the care provided.

When I met with the fostering team to discuss setting up the new group, the workers in the team described in a subtly contemptuous but overtly humorous way that running the monthly support group felt like facing 'a whinging and demanding mob' where they 'talk about nothing but grievances'. In that discussion, the social workers that ran it told me that each social worker in the fostering team took it in turn to run the group, and expressed extreme apprehension as their turn came around again. They used words like 'escaping', 'avoiding' and 'dreading' the encounters, and saw their role as chairing an unruly group, taking copious minutes and passing them on to a colleague who had the unenviable task of running it the following month.

Although I kept the thought to myself at the time, I noted they were describing a phenomenon whereby, rather than taking in or thinking about the strong and usually aggrieved feelings generated in and by the meeting, they wanted to get rid of the awful feelings by passing the baton quickly on to another social worker – mirroring the passing on of unmanageable children from one carer to the next in the form of placement breakdowns. Their descriptions echoed the words the foster carers used when describing the young people who they complained about: 'demanding', 'threatening', 'ungrateful' and 'never taking advice'.

The team supposed that because of our CAMHS perspective, we could provide specialist training so that the foster carers could learn how better to manage the difficult young people placed with them. Somehow, despite their own years of experience the CAMHS team was idealised with magic knowledge, while they were relegated to uselessness and stupidity. The more often the group overwhelmed each successive social worker, the more manic the behaviour was at the next one.

Holding horrible feelings

The hypothesis I presented was that many current and often 'manualised' foster or adoption parenting training courses, like the ones they were employing, presuppose a state of mind in the carers that is available for cognitive engagement, and that there was a willingness to take something in; in other words, being in a state of mind to access what was on offer, I was querying the capacity of some of the more overwhelmed foster carers to call upon the more thinking aspects of themselves. I was suggesting that the work they were doing, living with such disturbed and disturbing children, was figuratively rendering them 'learning dis-abled'. As a protection against the children's extreme behaviours and emotions, their own thinking was being replaced by concrete mental entities that cannot be explored. Bion (1959) describes this phenomenon, explaining how destroying links between thoughts allows one to fend off extreme anxiety that is proving literally unthinkable.

In our specialist CAMHS service for looked after and adopted children we were often referred young people who were emotionally overwhelmed and traumatised. They were often described in the referrals as 'unable to learn'. Concerned by a growing body of evidence that looked after children have poorer educational outcomes (NICE, 2013; DfE, 2010), there has been greater emphasis in govern-ment policy on educational achievement. Recent advances in neuroscience have also been valuable in identifying connections between learning difficulties and neurological impingement pre- and post-birth. But less attention has been paid to the emotional aspects of learning and thinking.

Bion (1967a) developed a theory which explored a particular aspect of the mother's care which helps the baby begin to process powerful and overwhelming emotional experiences. He suggested that the baby projects or evacuates raw emotions into the mother, who takes them in and processes them in her own mind, returning them to the baby in more digestible and bite-sized pieces. He called this capacity in the mother 'containment'. Over time the baby takes in this aspect of the mother's care and, by internalising it, is able to give meaning to its own emotional states. If a mother is unable to be emotionally available to her baby in this way there is no modification of these terrifying states of mind, which become what Bion described as a state of 'nameless dread'.

Destroying links between feelings and thoughts allows the baby to fend off 'nameless dread'. Not knowing is safer and less painful. This internal process of not putting thoughts together, of avoiding thought, can become a characteristic of the developing personality. What we know is that babies learn to think through a process of being empathetically thought about.

Faced with the foster children's defensive attacks on thinking, and filled up with the disturbing projections of the children placed in their care, why should we imagine that the foster carers can maintain a state of mind more available for thought and the making of meaning? In the same way that these children faced an early deficit in containment, foster carers are often suffering from a deficit of the containing function of the supervising social worker. This role in current practice through resource restrictions, austerity, and managerialism, has been depleted of its task of providing emotional support. The culture of social services departments have come to feel more persecutory; and the statutory requirement of imposing a more rigid tick-box 'assessment function' can generate in the foster carer/supervising social worker relationship feelings of being visited by a critical, judgemental and insensitive authority figure. Foster carers are increasingly left without help to process some of the more scary and traumatic experiences which are brought squarely into their homes while feeling more scrutinised and exposed.

> One foster carer told me, with much anger, how her social worker 'had not even bothered to take off her shoes and tracked filth and garbage all through the house!' Another had added, 'you should meet my new one … she's always trying to find some little thing wrong that she can get me on … how would she like it if I went snooping in her house?'

So the plan for the group was to offer a consistent, reliable and containing experience that would in time allow for the development of a 'thinking capacity'. If the anxieties could be contained, this in turn would allow the foster carers to 'take in' and use some specialist information and knowledge. Like abused and neglected children, 'taking in' – food, nurture, parental thoughts and feelings – could in fact be quite toxic, and the safer position is to turn away. But if the foster carers could have an experience of a stable supportive group they might be able to transfer that to the experience they offer to the children.

Therefore the group was designed as an experiential group, or what I have come to call a 'psycho-educational' model. Unlike social learning theory, which posits that learning is a cognitive process that takes place in a social context and can occur purely through observation or direct instruction (Bandura, 1977), experiential learning involves a direct encounter with the phenomena being studied rather than merely thinking about the encounter, or only considering the possibility of doing something about it. My role as group facilitator, like that Bion attributed to the maternal function, was to transform un-metabolised experience into thought and thinking. But first I had to bear it!

The nuts and bolts

On a practical basis, the group met once a fortnight for two hours, negotiated with difficulty to fit between what the carers described as other 'demands' like school runs and lunch duties. There was a closed membership, and it was planned to continue over the course of a year. I undertook to provide tea/coffee/biscuits and a consistent and comfortable room. The overall structure was intended to be an hour for more didactic input as required by the team manager and an hour for discussion focused on applying theoretical ideas to one of the foster children each week, allowing space for the group members to reflect and to support each other.

At the outset, I sent invitations to all of the local authority's foster carers. I assumed I would have sufficient requests and could offer an individual meeting to each carer in advance of the group starting, explaining the group and making an initial connection to each of the participants. The reality was quite different. There were no takers, and in the end, social workers were 'encouraging' the foster carers on their caseloads for whom there was the most concern or anxiety.

I did not meet the members until the first day, and most were not really sure what this 'training' group was for. There were 10 participants. They conveyed at the outset a feeling that, rather than attending by choice, membership was more akin to a court imposed care order (S31) than voluntary accommodation under S20 (Children Act, 1989). Further, in the inadvertent rush to set it up, the first encounter felt much like an emergency placement rather than a planned move.

There was an agreement that the discussion in the group would remain confidential unless there were issues of risk, but that I would share general themes with the fostering team at a termly review. Like with the children in their care, there was a complicated boundary between what was part of family life, and what needed to be shared with others.

In the beginning, the group felt completely unmanageable

Having already set out kettles and mugs and the makings of a snack, I would arrive in the room on time, where two or three foster carers would already have been brought by the receptionist. They would barely look up or stop their conversations, or one would try to grab my attention immediately with details of some dramatic incident in the week. When I actually managed to make a start with the group, the door would be opened and a further member would arrive, talking as they came in, calling out to other members who they already knew. This pattern of arriving, one at a time, over the first hour, without a sense that anything was going on until they got there puzzled me at first. I found myself feeling annoyed and unsettled at what felt like extreme and unacknowledged rudeness. Often the entrances felt dramatic, with some story of a terrible incident that had recently occurred with their foster child tumbling out of their mouths before they even sat down.

Early conversation veered toward social interactions, pulling everyone to discuss some TV show or current event. Alternatively, they would recount stories of recent 'useless' training events that they had been made to attend and revisit grievances about fostering allowances that were not paid, or requests denied or forgotten. It felt like a constant stream of criticism and complaint against the local authority, the social workers or the young people. Attempts on my part to engage them in discussions about the purpose of the group or topics of interest were quickly diverted, and my plan to give them each an opportunity to introduce themselves and their foster children to the group was avoided by some, while a few seemed to divulge very personal material. The tenor of the group was full of grievance. I quickly felt overwhelmed and out of my depth. In fact, I felt like what the foster carers must feel.

In the next few weeks, at their request for me to provide training on attachment theory, I came with a prepared hand-out. In fact it sat on my lap for the entire time as one foster carer after the other shared horrendous stories of the struggles they were having with a child in their care. Yet listening, I found the stories hard to follow and lost both the chronology and thread of the narrative.

> One of the foster carers came with a video on her phone of her foster child, wanting us to hear the stream of abusive language. She had, in a previous week, stood up and mimicked this girl in a humorous but rather denigratory way, complaining of the torrent of abuse she suffered. Another foster carer talked at length of how their young person never looked after anything and had managed to throw away or lose most of the cutlery in the house. This woman was irate that when she went to find a spoon for her coffee there were none left – 'she made it impossible for us to eat,' she said; and then she made the young person search the rubbish bin to find some of the spoons she had thrown away, threatening to take it out of her pocket money if she had to buy replacements. The young person had gone upstairs and trashed her room.

After a few weeks, driven by an increasing feeling that I was not offering the 'training' that the local authority was commissioning and that I would be criticised and the group ended when they got feedback, I suggested to the group members that they take the hand-outs and maybe have a chance to read them at home. Filled with my own anxiety, I fell back on trying to make them think, to impose knowledge on them, when they were clearly communicating that their experiences were attacking their ability to take in ideas. Not surprisingly then, over the next few weeks, they 'forgot' to read them, or even that they had been given something to read, while at the same time complaining that I was not teaching them anything, and that coming to the group was a waste of time.

Certainly something at that stage felt extremely primitive; I felt I was being faced with an undifferentiated cohort of critical, complaining and dissatisfied need – the 'demanding mob' that had been described by the supervising social work team. The chaos, the selfish presentation of some of the members (that the group only started to exist when they arrived) and the general over-dependence on false social interaction all seem to be both about the infantile nature of beginnings, while echoing the experience of the beginnings of a new placement. For them, the foster children must have felt like they were bursting into their homes, ignoring or conversely grabbing the carer's attention, imposing their own social rules, tossing opportunities to eat straight into the bin, and often full of grievance. Through projective identification, a defence mechanism that describes how what is unbearable is split off and evacuated into the mind of another in such a way that it has an impact on the other, I was being made to know what it feels like to be rubbish.

Klein (1946) explained that the tiny baby, before the infant mind is capable of complex thought, needs to rid itself of unsatisfactory, disturbing or bad feelings in order to protect good feelings. This entails the capacity to 'split' the good part of things from the bad part of things and then to send, or what she termed 'project', the bad feelings somewhere else to be rid of them. If you have ever been alongside a distressed and screaming baby, you will know how their distressed, anxious or frightened feelings affect you. It is this process that allows the baby to communicate its feelings to a receptive carer before it has the capacity for words or even thoughts. 'Bion found that people who have been deprived of emotional containment as a child project with great intensity when the opportunity is offered' (Bower, 2005: 11).

The British analyst, Denis Carpy (1989) added a further dimension to these ideas. He suggested that the baby not only projects but simultaneously observes the mother as she works to endure and understand the communication. As well as being contained the baby also observes whether the mother is able to survive the intensity of the bad feelings and how she is affected by the projections. According to him, some development of the baby's infantile mind takes place as a gradual process of identification with and introjection of the mother's mind and thinking capacity.

Certainly at this early stage of the group's development, I was being made to feel overwhelmed and inadequate. The foster carers were projecting the feelings of being useless into me, and then, on an unconscious level, watching how I coped with it.

The first step in early development is the establishment of a satisfying relationship between the baby and aspects of the mother's care; gazing, feeding, holding and cleaning. In time the baby establishes within its mind an image of this experience and the equivalents to these processes develop in the psyche. Feeding fundamentally sustains life while also establishing an emotional parallel of taking something in; pace, amount, satisfaction, timeliness, as well as a developing trust that what is being ingested is good and not toxic. Being held securely in parental arms, and the holding of the baby in parental minds, allows for the development in the baby of containment, while cleaning – nappy changing and onwards through to appropriate toilet training – has psychic equivalence first to getting rid of and managing the 'messy' feelings, and in time to controlling where and when the mess gets deposited.

Food and feeding

For many weeks, the manifest content of the group's discussions was often about food. Each week one of the carers would inevitably share a story about how a foster child would refuse to join their family for dinner, but later they would find dirty plates and hoarded food in their rooms. They would talk in detail about how they had tried to cook the right food (appropriate for the culture of the child) only to find that after all their effort, the child preferred fish fingers or McDonald's. The food their own families ate was often rejected, left unfinished on the table, scraped into the bins or spat out.

One week we heard how a foster child, described by her carer as 'greedy', ate continuously until she vomited. Another foster carer told how a seven-year-old had thrown a plate of food on their newly painted dining room wall. In great detail she described how the sauce had dripped down the wall like tears, while the boy laughed maniacally and refused to help clean it up when she remonstrated. There was a sense of triumph when she reported she had sent him to bed and told him to stay in his room. Some other members of the group shook their head in agreement with what they called her firm stance. The group ignored my idea that this might have been similar to what happened in his birth family.

The foster carers were throwing away the 'food for thought' that I was giving them – would I send them away? These stories about difficulties with feeding the children properly were often told with annoyance or worry that the child would complain to the LAC nurse or their social worker that they were not being fed and they would be accused of starving the child.

In the group, having supplied tea (both black and fruit) and coffee, I was often admonished by the group members for not having the right herb teas, or sweet-eners for anyone who had diabetes (no one actually did!). Each week I brought biscuits and fruit (the borough had a healthy eating policy) and often there were guarded comments about the biscuits and whether they should or should not have chocolate, or whether the fruit could or could not be eaten without needing a knife. I started to notice that, despite my invitation to help themselves, no one ate anything throughout the two hours, and then, when the group finished, the members would hang around talking to each other and pile napkins up with whatever was on the table, surreptitiously filling their handbags.

One member of the group, a woman I will refer to as Lorna, told us each week how well the 'difficult' child she was fostering was settling and what a good job she was doing compared to the child's two previous foster carers where there had been placement breakdowns. Often she would give advice to the others. Many times when I shared an idea or thought, Lorna would put forward her own views, which according to her, made much more sense than any suggestions I made.

One week on my way in, I stopped to pick up the milk and fruit, and noticed some seasonal plums, which I bought, feeling pleased that I was pro-viding something more special. During the group that week, while another woman, Jean, was telling us about how her foster child had been self-harming and I was clarifying aspects of risk, Lorna suddenly looked over at the fruit on the table and blurted out, 'those plums look just like the plums I bought this week'. She then got out of her chair, walked to the table and picked one up and took a bite. She chewed for a moment, and then very dramatically spat it into her hand making loud sounds of disapproval and disgust. Finally, she wrapped what remained in a napkin she retrieved from the table and tossed it like a basket ball player across the room into the rubbish bin, saying trium-phantly 'yuck – my plums were much better than those plums', and then returned to her seat and extolled Jean to carry on.

Klein (1984) introduced the idea of envy as the angry feelings that another person possesses and enjoys something else desirable, often accompanied by an impulse to take it away or spoil it. This attack on the special fruit I provided seemed an attack on my capacity to tolerate them better than they can tolerate the children.

In time, and through the use of supervision, I could make links in my mind. The competitive attacks on what I provided, my own desire to provide something special, the surreptitious rather than overt taking – almost hoarding – of the food to be eaten later in their own 'rooms': all of these were communications that I had to notice and take in. Yet the complexity and the ferocity of the projections often made understanding them in the moment impossible.

Evacuation and communication through impact

One member, Margaret, a first-time foster carer managing her first placement of three young traumatised refugee siblings, would brightly say each week how much she enjoyed coming to the group and meeting the other carers and how much she looked forward to it. She clearly felt sympathetic to the children in her care, despite the problems she was having, particularly with the youngest who suffered from encopresis and defecated in his pants regularly. She described in an animated voice how she was always cleaning him, cleaning the mess up, and even having to go into school to help them manage. At first she presented as coping well with this awful situation, but in time her story had a less sympathetic quality and there was a more brittle tone. With each passing week, there was an added note of frustration and annoyance as she related stories about how difficult it was to get any one to help him or make him stop the behaviour, that no one was taking the problem seriously or doing anything, and it felt like she was talking to a wall. Each week, she repeated the story, adding a further complaint – but not ever leaving time for the group to discuss the incidents she was relaying. The detail in the narratives was often hard to follow and seemed each week to have a bit more embellishment. Eventually one week she came looking tired, almost 'shell shocked', and told us that it had transpired that the youngest boy had hepatitis C – and it had not been picked up in the initial medical! She explained in a rather detached manner how her grandchildren often stayed with her, and how she was now worried and needed to get them medically checked. The rest of the group grew irate – loudly berating the local authority, the health professionals, the social workers; giving opinions and advice.

Finally, after a few months, Margaret did not arrive at the group. (She was often early.) About fifty minutes later, in the middle of a discussion about how useless the safeguarding training many of them had attended the previous week was, the door slammed open and Margaret was standing in the doorway. She didn't say anything, but in her hand was a small packet containing photographs that she appeared to have collected from the chemist. Without a word, she handed it to one of the members, who looked through the photos and silently handed them to the person sitting next to her. This was repeated until the photos had made the rounds of the room finishing with me. There were a dozen photos of excrement! There was a pile on a pristine parquet floor, a pile on a lovingly crocheted coverlet on a bed, a pile on the top of a basket of clean laundry; literally there was a pile of shit. It was shocking – the defiling of immaculate objects with such a mess.

There was a shocked silence in the room for a while. Finally Margaret sat down and quietly started to weep.

Coming away from this session, it took me a while to gather my own thoughts. I felt angry and sad. It was difficult not to join in the group's anger, blaming the social worker for not having known that the boy had hepatitis; or being angry with the birth family for their lack of care. My struggle not to join their anger and despair and to survive the intensity of the bad feelings will have been observed by the group. So what was Margaret's behaviour actually about, and what explains the move from grievance to grief?

It must have felt to Margaret as if, despite her attempts to communicate the horror of her experience, that the group was impervious and unwilling to take in her awful feelings. She was unconsciously invited to join the psychic retreat of the group, to join the aggrieved state, to protect from the pain and vulnerability. Learning about the hepatitis C, the risk she had unwittingly exposed her own grandchildren to, had overwhelmed her original capacity to cope. Exposed to an event that she could not digest, and without the adequate containment from her support network, either her daughter, who was angry with her for the risk to her children, or from the professionals whose role it was to support her, she posited her messy feelings into the group in a concrete way – through photographs – in much the way the foster child evacuated his mess on her. As a new foster carer, her initial hope to use the group as a container was thwarted by a membership of 'experienced' carers who had long since built up impermeable defences when they had not been contained.

Margaret's experience, that the group had finally, through seeing the photographs, really taken in the horror and pain of the child and her own terror at exposing her family to hepatitis, resulted in her being able to be in touch with the feelings and relinquish her aggrieved state of mind. She was finally able to cry.

Certainly she had reason to complain, as did many of the carers about their own experiences. What distinguishes a grievance from a complaint, however, is what Betty Joseph (1982) describes as the extent of the hostility, and the perverse gratification derived from 'repetitive ruminations'. In her view, the aggrieved person is caught in an addictive yet gratifying internal dynamic of accusing and blaming in a way that represents a destructive attack on themselves or on attempts at help. Aggrieved people can appear to helping professionals to prefer grumbling monotonously to engaging in changing something. Peter Blos (1991) described how the aggrieved client comes to view him or herself as a victim and acts as if the professional or therapist is the perpetrator, inflicting the pain through their interventions.

Looked after children often come into care following neglect or abuse. In the external as well as the internal world, they do not have full access to a mother – both as part of the neglect of the early years and as a result of being in care. Those experiences feel and *are* unjust and can be unbearable and are often managed through controlling and omnipotent behaviour.

In this way we can begin to think about grievance in both the children and the foster carers as a possible response to trauma, where the repetitive complaint offers some gratification in itself. Interventions that might help with grieving, part of the ordinary emotional work necessary to manage loss and trauma, are rejected so that the grievance can continue protecting against the feelings of pain. This conversion of hurt to anger might be more helpfully understood as an unconscious defensive strategy to avoid feelings of helplessness or powerlessness while the repetitive quality traps the aggrieved person into not knowing about their own distress.

Throughout those first months the group had continued to feel unmanageable. Each week, someone in the group would complain that nothing was getting better, or that they were not learning anything, or that it was a waste of time coming and they had better things to do with their morning. Yet each week, when the two hours finished and I ended the session, most of the group stayed on chatting to each other, or individuals would attempt to engage me with some specific question. Despite their words to the contrary, it often felt like I had to 'push them out' of the room against their wishes. And each week, after the room was emptied, our kind team administrator, having hovered until they were gone, would come in and start to clear up the room, gathering things and taking them into the kitchenette. Looking at my exhausted face, she would 'shush' me out of the room, and after a gesture at helping her by limply carrying some mugs to the kitchen, I would gratefully retire to the team room where a colleague, knowing how I was struggling with the group, would ask how it went and offer to get me lunch or paracetamol. Each week after those early sessions, I would suffer from a splitting headache and feel exhausted and depleted. The group's emotional distress, pain and rage, defended against and unable to be thought about, got projected into me literally as a pain in my mind – a splitting headache. If experiences cannot be processed in the mind, then they can come to be somatised or experienced in the body.

The role of administrative staff in services for deprived people cannot be overestimated. Social workers are often the receptacles of 'shit' unbearable feelings. Being practically cared for makes the job easier.

Acknowledging secondary trauma: progress is made

The session after the Christmas break started with the usual social interactions. They started to share holiday stories. Many complained about the behaviours of their foster children during the school break, and the lack of planning by the social workers for birth family contact. A rather quiet member who had previously seemed unable to find a voice, said loudly to me as the group was assembling: 'welcome back. We thought you might have stayed in NY and never returned!'

Without thinking, I smiled and said that I had thought about it, 'but you couldn't get rid of me that easily!' Something slightly shifted. Perhaps I had finally conveyed that I was staying put and could withstand their projection.

For the first time since we began to meet it felt like they might be able to take in some new ideas. Later that session, a more quiet member, Sara, told the group about her foster child who had kept her awake with nightmares and screaming throughout the holidays following a contact visit. Then Sara continued by telling us that she was exhausted, and described how even after the child was finally asleep, she also had nightmares of being trapped in a dark cellar with vermin, which woke her, and she couldn't get back to sleep. There seemed actually to be a pause as I made a link between the child's nightmares and Sara's.

The word trauma was originally used by Freud (1920) as a metaphor to explain how the mind can be pierced and wounded by events. Current developments in neuroscience have helped us to further understand that the mind must selectively shut out excessive amounts and kinds of stimulation to be able to function. For infants and young children in ordinary circumstances that filtering function is largely served by the mother or primary carer though her sensitivity to what her baby is able to manage at any particular time. A primary carer is meant to protect the baby from the extremes of experience, both environmental and emotional. A neglected or abused child is deprived of that parental filter and, without the experience of a containing parental mind, is exposed to what we have come to call early relational trauma – when the same person who is meant to be protecting it inflicts the wound on the child. In adulthood, people who have had a sufficient and appropriate parental shield will have built up inside themselves a capacity to manage this filtering themselves. Those who have not can be more vulnerable.

Not all terrible events must be traumatic. For an experience to really be a trauma, the event must break through the filtering process and override the ordinary emotional strategies that have developed to allow that person to cope with difficulties. The trauma occurs when the mind is flooded with a kind and degree of stimulation that is far more than it can make sense of or manage. For the child's immature mind, it means that there is also no parental mind available to help. Something very violent feels as though it has happened internally, and this mirrors the violence that is felt to have happened, or indeed has happened in the external world.

Foster carers, exposed regularly and sometimes continuously to the young person's behaviour (the child's vivid recounting of their abuse, for example, or when awakened by the child's nightmares and night terrors and going to comfort them, or during observation of the intrusive thoughts), are by extension witnessing the traumatic events too. Without suitable support and containment, the foster carer is suffering the same exposure to the events without helpful filtering and is being traumatised themselves. This phenomenon has come to be called secondary trauma.

Originally thought about in respect of professionals and therapists working with patients suffering PTSD, a foster carer's proximity to a looked after child who is in care due to early relational trauma means that she is exposed 24/7 to that child's traumatic presentation in intimate and inescapable ways. The foster carer's subsequent cognitive or emotional representation of that event may result in a set of symptoms and reactions that parallel PTSD.

Some foster carers have successful networks of support, either personal or professional. Supervising social workers historically offered mitigation against the trauma through regular, consistent and benign visits where thinking about the experience was possible. However, in contemporary fostering practice, there are often very limited resources to help foster carers process this experience for themselves or to think about the experiences of the looked after children who are living with them.

Exposure to someone with unprocessed trauma is not only like experiencing the trauma, but can re-awaken primary trauma. Therefore proximity to traumatised children and young people can sometimes re-awaken earlier losses in the carers. Some foster carers have been separated from their own parents without the necessary attunement of other adults, or may have unresolved experiences of abuse or neglect themselves. It is a long held belief in social care that once the carer can tell you about their experiences they have 'resolved' them. However, this may be a misunderstanding. The retelling of a personal narrative in a repetitive, fragmented or manic way might be a symptom of a trauma rather than evidence of the processing of it.

In sharing my 'understanding' of secondary trauma, the group finally felt more interested and engaged. Giving their experiences a name and a reason, making links between their feelings and the children's, seemed to shift the discussion from the concrete recounting of their awful experiences, to something more reflective.

As the months followed there was less reliance on relating grievances and repetitive vignettes of awful behaviour. When they did tell the story there was more opportunity to think about what the behaviour might be about and there was some interest in what thinking I could provide. A few said they would pause after something bad had happened with the foster child, and say to themselves, 'what would Robin say?' For a while they needed to share my mind, to introject a containing Robin/carer, before their own capacity to think under fire developed. By this time their stories usually had more coherence, and group members could make some links between the different behaviours of their foster children. It felt like there was less blame. I was amazed to hear them describe a much wider range of emotions. The children were less demonised and they seemed to feel relief that their own feelings might be affected by the exposure to the children's trauma.

The months passed and we were beginning to near the end of the group. I often spoke about when we would be finishing and how many more sessions we had. Some members of the group expressed concern about how they would manage when the group finished. At one point some members demanded that the group carry on, and there was a period where this got expressed as a grievance against social services who they depicted as withholding further sessions. The tendency to idealise the group took hold. Yet overall, there was more of an acceptance that they had actually had a good 'feed' and were understood. The ending came with sadness but not grievance. They had more sense that there were other ways to gain sustenance.

Supervision and the couple relationship

From the beginning and built into the psycho-educational model was the requirement for supervision, built in as a reliable container. My manager, psychoanalytically trained, provided regular fortnightly consultation. Faced with projections of aggrieved, traumatised foster carers, supervision provided a partnership; a 'parental' couple who could put their heads together to think through the disturbance and help to enable the capacity to keep one's mind in the face of attacks against thinking. In the same way that the maternal mind can be overwhelmed in the early days after birth by both their own and the baby's feelings and needs the containment of a second carer, so I needed to be joined in a 'parental couple' to manage to process the enormity of the group's emotional state.

I undertook to write detailed process notes about each group session. After the first session I set about writing up my notes only to find that I could barely remember anything. Fragments of what people said got merged with moments of observation. I found it difficult to differentiate between the members and I could not articulate my own feelings properly. In the end I had lots of bullet points but no sentences. There were coffee stains where my cup had spilled over the rim as I tried to read what came out of the printer.

Arriving for that first supervision I felt stupid, exposed and ashamed. Despite so many years of experience, how could I have apparently achieved so little and remembered less. I felt a fraud, in tears. My mind invested in my supervisor all the knowledge, while I felt useless. We spent that first session knowing together about a mind that could not think. She held on to the belief that there was a way to understand this.

In time, my process notes grew longer and more coherent. I could think about the group, at least in hindsight. In the group however, throughout those first months, keeping my thinking mind remained difficult. At times I literally brought her with me by mentioning her name, almost as a way of validating my thoughts. I found myself saying that 'Becky [not her real name] and I think' or 'when Becky and I were thinking about the group last week, we thought …'

In the latter stages of the group, although supervision continued, concretely bringing Becky with me into the group room became less necessary. My own mind seemed more able to filter out and let in. I felt I could take in and digest more while in the group. As the group's projections diminished, I was less defensive and could use my mind for thinking.

So what was I to make of this group?

Psychoanalytic ideas might help to explain some of what might otherwise have felt like extraordinarily rude, inappropriate and 'unprofessional' behaviour. Without a way to understand it and someone to join me in that endeavour, I might easily have responded by getting caught up in unhelpful enactments or by retaliating and returning the terrible feelings that were being projected into me.

As described previously, feeding and evacuating, the taking in of or failing to take in mental and emotional experiences happens through processes of introjection and projection (Klein, 1959). In this way, the baby can rid its mind of unsatisfactory, disturbing or bad experiences. This entails the capacity to 'split' the good part of things from the bad parts of things, and to 'send' (project) the bad feelings somewhere else. Bion (1967b) stressed that the development of the capacity to think and to 'digest' emotional experiences is a result of a containing maternal function. He is describing the primary caregiver's capacity to bear the psychically immature infant's overwhelming sensations and feelings. In this process, the primary parent needs to make mental space for the particular infant and its unique cues. The parent struggles to make sense of her baby's needs and distress through attentive observation, exploration and thinking. The infant's non-integrated, sometimes overwhelming feelings, projected into the parent, are thus contained or 'digested' and transformed into tolerable mental content before being fed back to the infant. An emotionally available caregiver is able to attend to and make sense of her baby's communications and then, through her behaviours, give the baby an experience of having been understood.

In 'feeding', much as a parent bird needs to first chew the worm, adding its own enzymes so as to pre-digest it and then feed it to its chick in a more manageable form, the early parental function of 'containment' supplies the infant with a healthy emotional environment in which to develop the capacity to manage its own feelings. In this way, the baby internalises not only the metabolised content but also the capacity to tolerate, think about and mentally contain its own experiences. My main function as the group facilitator was to provide an equivalent containing function.

As a result of early abuse and neglect, requisite mental digestion and containment for the children in care have been disrupted and distorted. It is no coincidence that the foster carers in the group were often pre-occupied by the difficulties in feeding the foster children – both literally and metaphorically. As a mirror to this, they were simultaneously refusing my attempts either to digest their communications or feed them with any thoughts or 'training food'.

Often group members would speak at great length telling disturbing narratives about their foster children. Unlike some telling of stories, which can feel like a relief, these stories were often repetitive and told in unsympathetic terms or in flat or angry voices. This attempt to evacuate the feelings felt more like a way to be rid of them rather than think about them. My early attempts to 'digest' and make meaning out of these stories and feelings felt inadequate. What I had to take in felt overwhelming. Moreover there seemed to be little sense in the group that I had heard or really understood the horror of their experiences.

Further to Freud and Klein, some later analytic theorists have suggested that one of the most valuable aspects of projective identification, as well as its intended purpose of communication by impact, is to allow the patient (or in this case the foster carers group) to unconsciously watch the recipient to see how they manage. Stark gathers ideas from these later theorists to help explain.

> It has been proposed (Carpy, 1989, Pick, 1985) that, paradoxically, part of what makes projective identification so effective is the fact that the therapist can never completely contain what the patient projects into her and in fact, may well have to struggle to contain it at all. In other words, the therapist will often partially act out her countertransference, which as Irma Brenman Pick

(1985) has hypothesized, allows the patient to see that the therapist (1) is affected by what the patient has projected into her; (2) must struggle to tolerate it; but (3) ultimately manages to contain it without grossly acting it out. Carpy (1989) hypothesizes that it is through this process that the patient is able gradually to re-internalize previously unmanageable aspects of herself. Particularly transformative is the patient's recognition of the therapist's capacity – despite her struggle – to tolerate the patient's toxic parts.

(Stark, 2000: 275)

It is important to understand how things get acted out if they cannot be thought about. For example, although the foster carers could talk about how the children would not take their food or take in their help, this was rendered meaningless until they enacted this phenomenon by not taking in, denigrating or sneaking off with my biscuits and fruit while experiencing my capacity not to criticise or retaliate but rather to struggle to make links between their stories and these actions. Towards the end they no longer had to turn away from my 'metaphorical food' – the thoughts and making meaning. Their exposure to trauma was noticed, so their defences against the pain could diminish sufficiently to find the group valuable.

The fostering team, unable to tolerate the experience of being on the receiving end of so much grief and grievance without this understanding and without the necessary supervision, had quickly passed along the facilitation of the 'support group' – handing over the 'minutes' but not holding the experience, much in the same way that the foster carers could not bear the grief and disturbance of the children and quickly passed them on, with their files, to other foster carers in the form of a placement breakdown.

A foster carer's job is to experience the projections of looked after infants and children and contain/digest them until they can help to put them into words. I needed to process in myself a disturbing, disrupting and anti-educational process. Unless this is understood, training and support groups for foster carers can feel like failures.

Afterword

The illustrations given have been anonymised and are amalgams from different groups that were run over a number of years and under the auspices of different local authorities. At the outset of each group we asked each carer to fill out strength and difficulties questionnaires (SDQs) for each child and a second questionnaire about their experiences as foster carers. In follow-ups after each group, while the SDQs for the children remained the same, the foster carers reported feeling better able to manage the children. The social workers reported a parallel reduction in placement breakdowns during the life of the groups.

Acknowledgements

I would like to thank all of these unnamed foster carers and managers for their contributions to this learning.

References

Bandura, A. (1977) *Social Learning Theory*. Englewood Cliffs: Prentice Hall.

Bazalgette, L., Rahilly, T. and Trevelyan, G. (2015) *Achieving Emotional Wellbeing for Looked After Children*. London: NSPCC.

Bion, W.R. (1959) Attacks on linking. *International Journal of Psycho-Analysis* 40. Reprinted in (1967) *Second Thoughts*. London: Heinemann.

Bion, W.R. (1967a) A theory of thinking. In *Second Thoughts*. London: Heinemann.

Bion, W.R. (1967b) *Learning From Experience*. London: Heinemann.

Blos, P. (1991) Sadomasochism and the defence against recall of painful affect. *Journal of the American Psychoanalytic Association* 39(2), 417–429.

Bower, M. (2005) *Psychoanalytic Theory for Social Work Practice: Thinking Under Fire*. London: Routledge.

Carpy, Denis V. (1989) Tolerating the countertransference: a mutative process. *The International Journal of Psychoanalysis* 70(2), 287–294.

DfE (2010) *Promoting the Educational Achievement of Looked After Children: Statutory Guidance for Local Authorities*. Available from: www.dcsf.gov.uk [accessed 6 February 2017].

Freud, S. (1920) Beyond the pleasure principle. *Standard Edition* 18. London: Hogarth Press.

Joseph, B. (1982) Addiction to near death. *International Journal of Psychoanalysis* 63(4), 449–456.

Klein, M. (1946) Notes on some schizoid mechanisms. *International Journal of Psychoanalysis* 27, 99–110.

Klein, M. (1959) Our adult world and its roots in infancy. In (1975) *The Writings of Melanie Klein Vol.3*. London: Routledge.

Klein, M. (1984). *Envy and Gratitude and Other Works 1946–1963*. London: The Hogarth Press.

Munro, E. and Hardy, A. (2006) *Placement Stability: A Review of the Literature*. Loughborough: Loughborough University Press.

NICE (2013) *Quality Standard [QS31] for the Health and Wellbeing of Looked-After Children and Young People: Tailored Resource for Corporate Parents and Providers on Health and Wellbeing of Looked-After Children and Young People*. London: NICE.

Pick, I.J. (1985) Working through in the countertransference. *International Journal of Psychoanalysis* 66, 157–166.

Rock, S., Michelson, D., Thomson, S. and Day, C. (2015) Understanding foster placement instability for looked after children: a systematic review and narrative synthesis of quantitative and qualitative evidence. *British Journal of Social Work* 45 (1), 177–203.

Sinclair, I., Baker, C., Lee, J. and Gibbs, I. (2007) *The Pursuit of Permanence: A Study of the English Child Care System*. London: Jessica Kingsley Publishers.

Stark, M. (2000) *Modes of Therapeutic Action*. Northvale: Jason Aronson.

11

CRUEL PROTECTORS

Understanding sexual exploitation

Marion Bower and Robin Solomon

One of the difficulties of understanding sexual exploitation is that some aspects go against common sense. Professor Harry Ferguson summarises a case of exploitation from the newspapers. A girl of twelve or thirteen was taken to some woods and raped by seven men as a 'punishment'. Afterwards she was left alone, hurt and naked. However she did have her mobile phone. She did not ring her parents, social worker, police or ambulance. She rang one of the men who had just raped her. This is not an isolated case. *In fact one of the characteristics of many of these cases is the unwillingness of the girls to be rescued from their abusers*. This phenomenon is very similar to another social work experience: children who have been abused and neglected, and taken into care, may run away from kind foster parents back to their abusive families.

To understand this we need to learn why some young women are drawn to men who will treat them in an abusive way. Reports indicate that the presents used to groom the girls are very small. Cinema tickets, a DVD, a milkshake. Common sense would suggest these girls are seeking attention. The question is what sort of attention are they *unconsciously* seeking.

Many of the victims of sexual exploitation have been in care or are known to social services. The bar for coming into care these days is set very high: parental drug abuse, child sexual abuse and serious parental mental health problems. There is a wish to believe that coming into care makes children 'safe'. In fact they are carrying the scars of their early experiences. One of the things that they have often lost is the capacity to distinguish between good and bad experiences and people.

Freud's early work led him to discover that young children have sexual feelings, which he characterised as oral, anal and genital. These eventually gave way to adult sexuality. At first Freud thought that sexual abuse was widespread because so many patients reported it. Later he attributed these reports to fantasy. Unfortunately he threw the baby out with the bathwater. We now know that sexual abuse of children by adults is widespread. Many young people in the care system have been sexually abused. The consequences of this are complex. Some research by Judith Trowell and her colleagues (Long, Trowell and Miles, 2005) had two very relevant findings. The girls studied were aged nine to 13. All had experienced 'contact abuse', often by a father. One group of girls were allocated weekly psychotherapy, and the parents or carers were offered support. The researchers expected the girls to be preoccupied by the abuser, but they were instead preoccupied by *an unavailable mother*. One girl tried repeatedly to put a baby doll in a mother doll's arms, but it dropped. The girl tried over and over. Eventually she gave up and the dolls were made to engage in sexualised play. (This figure of a mother who turns a blind eye seems to be replicated in the professional networks.) For some girls it was the father, even if he was the abuser, who was felt to be the available parent. One girl said that all their pets had died since their father had gone to prison, as he was the only one who had looked after them. Many of the girls played and used their bodies in a highly sexualised way. Freud would have referred to this as *repetition compulsion*. He saw this as a way to master trauma by re-encountering and recreating it. Girls like this are of course easy prey for sexual exploitation.

Yasmin, aged 13, is the only child of a Moroccan mother and a Scottish father. Father is a heavy drinker and sometimes beats up mother. Yasmin came to the attention of social services when she was ten. She rarely appeared in school and it was discovered that she was being kept at home in bed with her mother. It was suspected that the mother sexually abused her, but nothing could be proved. A social worker began taking her into school. Yasmin told her class teacher that her father made her watch a snuff movie, a pornographic film where the woman is killed. She was very upset and was taken into care. She was placed with a foster mother where she was the only child. She refused to see her parents. In secondary school Yasmin started hanging out with a group of older boys. It was suspected that she was having sex with them. Yasmin refused to talk about this. Her old social worker had left and a new one saw her less often. The foster carer had a younger child placed with her, who needed a lot of attention. For a week Yasmin went to see the school counsellor every day, but sat in silence. At the end of the week Yasmin walked in front of a train and was killed.

How are we to understand this? Yasmin was brought up in a family where there was no clearly good or helpful parent. As she grew older she realised her parents lied to her to turn her against people who tried to help her. Once she was in care she refused to see her parents. This made her more dependent on her social worker and foster mother. When her social worker left and her foster mother was preoccupied with a younger child she must have felt angry and abandoned. The wish to kill herself came from a psychotic part of her personality which frightened her – her daily visits to the school counsellor were an unrecognised cry for help.

Yasmin's parents trapped her in a crazy world where they co-opted Yasmin into perverse activity, which probably defended the parents against psychotic breakdown. Yasmin's social worker and foster carer tried to engage her in the real world. However she retreated from this into sexual risk-taking with older boys.

Yasmin did not have trustworthy, good figures in her own mind, so she could not tolerate her social worker leaving or her foster carer becoming busy. With a less traumatic history her sexual risk-taking might have held her together. However, what actually happened is that she descended into a psychotic breakdown and killed herself.

Yasmin's case is a very extreme one. The crucial factors seem to be whether or not a young person has an internal world of good people who can be trusted. Melanie Klein describes an early stage in the baby's development which help it sort out good and bad people. She found that from the beginning of life a baby seeks contact with her mother (or other). The baby wants to take in good things and get rid of bad things through the mechanisms of introjection (taking in) and projection. These are psychological processes which reflect the physical processes of eating and excreting. Initially the mother is felt to be either very good or very bad. Some of the mother's 'badness' is amplified if the baby projects its own aggression into the mother. This is *projective identification*. Klein called this stage of development 'the paranoid schizoid position'. This early state of mind is very important because it enables us to distinguish 'good' from 'bad'. It is very important that there is in reality a caring, loving mother. Part of the role of a helpful mother is not simply to be present for the baby but to help it process difficult experiences. Wilfred Bion, one of Klein's most talented patients, suggested that the baby projects unbearable emotions into the mother. The mother processes them in her own mind and returns them to her baby in a more bearable form. The baby also internalises the mother's capacity for *containment*. Yasmin, in the example above, did not have a mother she could project into. Instead her mother used her as a receptacle for her own disturbing ideas. This capacity for containment, which is part of the persona of a good mother, helps the baby and, later, the child regulate difficult feelings.

At the time we began to write this chapter, when there seemed to be an absolute epidemic of sexual exploitation, an extraordinarily apt play was having a hit on the London stage. It was a dramatisation of an eighteenth-century novel written in letter form, *Les Liaisons Dangereuses*. It has also been made into at least two successful films, so it must speak to us now. It is a story of revenge and corruption. Cecile is a young girl who has been brought up in a convent. Her mother takes her out only to marry her off to an older man. Two bored, amoral aristocrats, the Duc de Valmont and Madame Merteuil, agree that Valmont will seduce and corrupt Cecile so that her forthcoming marriage will be ruined, and they will have their revenge on Cecile's mother. Valmont does this and Cecile becomes enslaved by him, even though the violence of their sex has killed their unborn baby. Cecile also rejects a kind and honourable suitor. The book does not draw attention to this, but one factor which makes Cecile vulnerable is that she has had a loveless upbringing in the convent. Cecile's mother is only interested in her to marry her off. There are no good people, only Cecile's rejected suitor.

Some of this pattern is repeated in real life case material. Linda was fifteen. She lived with a single mother who was depressed. Her parents separated when she was small and she had no contact with her father. At a club she met a musician who was ten years older. She had sex with him, even though she knew he slept with other women. She contracted salpingitis (an infection of the fallopian tubes). She delayed getting help until it had spread, and she was told she might be infertile. Despite her mother's attempts to stop her she continued to sleep with the musician. She was now sixteen. When Linda's mother spoke to social services, she was told that it was a 'lifestyle choice'. This expression is sometimes used about girls who have been in care, but turn to prostitution.

Both Linda and Cecile do not seem to have been abused, so why do they turn to abusive men? *We do not believe that turning to abusive men is a choice for these girls, it is an addiction.* It is used to defend the mind against feelings which would otherwise be felt to be intolerable. Once the girls have become involved in this, guilt about the damage to their bodies is added to their emotional pain. This helps us understand why victims of sexual exploitation return repeatedly to their abusers. Once the abuse stops they have to face the damage to themselves and their lives. It is very difficult to talk of this dynamic because of the risk of seeming to criticise the victims. However this has to be faced when designing treatment.

When a child or young person does not have the capacity to manage painful feelings they develop psychological defences which are extremely powerful. The psychoanalyst Herbert Rosenfeld (1971) describes a defensive organisation he calls 'the Mafia'. In this process omnipotent parts of the personality offer 'protection' to vulnerable, needy parts of the self. The price of 'protection' is that you are not allowed to leave the gang. Rosenfeld makes a distinction between the 'good' dependent self and the 'bad' omnipotent one. However a more disturbing and, we feel, more truthful version of this defence is given by the psychoanalyst John Steiner (1993). He suggests that instead of a clear-cut 'good' and 'bad' part of the self there is a sadomasochistic relationship between parts of the self. If we move this dynamic into the external world we can say that the girls carry the men's vulnerability and the men carry the girls' cruelty. The projective identification involved in this relationship leads to the situation described in the first paragraph of this chapter where the raped girl turns to one of her rapists for help. This link between abuser and abused is also enacted in one instance where some girls were raped in an underground car park. Afterwards the perpetrators wrote their own initials and those of the girls on the car park walls – rather like lovers carving their initials in a tree. (Afterwards the rapists tried to wash the evidence off the walls.)

A perpetrator

Unfortunately there is little in-depth knowledge about the sexual exploiters. We feel they should be treated by the full weight of the law, but understanding them might lead to prevention.

Gerry, aged 13, was referred to his local child guidance clinic for setting fire to his girlfriend's hair. He was brought to a clinic by his mother and stepfather. Gerry and his mother both looked angelic, whereas his stepfather was tall with a shaven head and seemed to have a knuckleduster on one hand. Gerry's mother, Mrs G, said Gerry was turning out exactly like his father (from whom she was divorced). Mrs G described how on two occasions Gerry's father had raped her while she was pregnant leading to two miscarriages. When Gerry heard this he started to cry. Mother and stepfather laid into him viciously calling him a wimp and other names. Gerry drew a picture of two big sharks and a little one 'in a tropical lagoon'. The little shark had dots beneath his eyes. I said 'are those tears?' Gerry said 'no, blood'. [I think tears were like blood to a shark for mother and stepfather.] Mrs G said that perhaps she would get Gerry's father to punish him. Gerry went white with fear. I felt paralysed and unable to challenge mother. Before he left Gerry said he did not want to come again, 'you just want to make me feel guilty'.

We can see what a disturbing environment Gerry has grown up in. His mother is the victim of a violent father, but at the same time she treats Gerry sadistically by threatening to get his father to punish him. We subsequently found out that when Gerry's father refused to punish him, Mrs G punched Gerry in the face so viciously that he was referred to social services. We would hypothesise that sexual exploiters come from families like this, where cruelty is idealised, vulnerability is attacked and the group is held together by the glue of sexual perversion. Newspaper reports make it clear that some exploiters come from the same families.

Turning a blind eye

One of the shocking aspects of the various reports on sexual exploitation is the way in which professionals, including the police and social services, turned a blind eye to what was well known. It is not enough to castigate professionals for this; we need to understand how it came about. The first thing we can say is that someone turning a blind eye is almost invariably a feature of sexual abuse. More commonly it is the mother. While sexual abuse is not identical to sexual exploitation, accounts from Rotherham, Oxford and elsewhere leave one asking 'where was the mother, police, or social services?' This is not a new phenomenon. In Sophocles's play *Oedipus Tyrannos*, written approximately 2500 years ago, the oracle at Delphi predicts he will kill his father and mother, Laius and Jocasta, King and Queen of Thebes. His parents send him away to be exposed on a mountain and die. However, the shepherd sent to do this gives him to another king and queen, who bring him up as their own child. When Oedipus hears the oracle he leaves his parents' home at once and sets off for Thebes. On the way there he meets his father, gets into a fight and kills him. The city of Thebes is being terrorised by the Sphinx. Oedipus is able to answer her riddle and she leaves. The prize is marrying Jocasta (his mother). The play makes clear that the citizens of Thebes probably have evidence of who Oedipus really is, and Jocasta must recognise the scars on his feet. Everyone turns a blind eye for the sake of political convenience. When Oedipus is forced to face the truth he puts out his own eyes. His mother hangs herself.

We have tried to show that the psychological consequences of giving up sexual exploitation is a psychic catastrophe. Interviews with victims show that they are in a bad way, often suffering from depression. It is assumed that this is because of the exploitation. We would suggest that it is because *the exploitation has stopped*. The fear of this psychic catastrophe gets into the professional networks. In Oedipus there is a fear of political instability which leads the citizens to turn a blind eye.

A similar point is made by Jane Milton, a psychiatrist and psychoanalyst who has worked with victims of physical and sexual abuse. These women often treat their own bodies and their children in cruel and perverse ways as a psychological defence against psychotic breakdown (Milton, 1994). She suggests that psychological improvement may lead to breakdown, and that victims should only be treated if there is intensive support available. The implications of this are very significant and there is an urgent need for research on the aftermath of sexual exploitation.

In the second part of this chapter, we look at some of the research into responses to sexual exploitation, and examine what happens in a situation where the professionals try *not* to turn a blind eye.

Professional responses

> As early as 1893 Freud drew attention to a state of mind that he described as 'blindness of the seeing eye', in which 'one knows and does not know a thing at the same time'.
>
> *(Britton, 1994: 1)*

While complete denial of reality was an indicator of a more psychotic state, Freud was describing a non-psychotic form of denial later termed *disavowal*. This was developed into the idea that unlike psychotic denial, disavowal obliterates only the significance of things, not their perception (Basch, 1983; Britton, 1994).

Thus we read about some professionals who, actually knowing about the horrible reality of the sexual exploitation of a young person in their care, wiped out the guilt and awful feelings by justifying their inability to keep the young people safe as 'respecting the young person's wishes and feelings', because that young person has said repeatedly that they want to return to the abusers. In fact the disavowal is the obliteration of the significance of the abuse, because the young person was thought of as an active participant, as wanting to take part.

A series of enquiries into child sexual exploitation makes this clear. In August 2014 Professor Alexis Jay published a review of child exploitation in Rotherham. It showed that organised sexual exploitation had been happening on a massive scale over many years. Local agencies had *dismissed concerns or put in place inadequate responses*. Shockingly, Louise Casey's report of February 2016 showed that, since the Jay report, many in the council and its local partners had continued to deny the scale of the problem, and not enough actions had been taken to stop the abuse. The government's white paper *Tackling Child Sexual Exploitation March 2015* lists 59 commitments including 'we will eradicate this culture of denial'.

The plans, while laudable, consist mostly of resources and education – 'alerting', 'funding' and 'training' (Home Office, 2015), while setting up structures meant to aid in the exchange of information and concerns. We believe that unless there is an understanding of how this culture of denial arises then it will be impossible to eradicate. No one seems to ask why otherwise competent police, social workers and health staff could not see what was in front of their noses, and denied it when directly challenged. Phrases like 'wishes and feelings of the child', intended to protect, can be perversely misused to do nothing.

A consultation to a children's home

In the first part of this chapter, we discussed the sado-masochistic dynamics of the victims and perpetrators, and the state of mind of the carers that participated, as well in the dynamics with the turning of a blind eye. We would now like to go on to think about why the professional networks around the young people were similarly dismissive and inadequate; and, reflecting the internal worlds of the young people themselves, denigrated their own capacity to help, and denied the serious-ness of the behaviour itself, thus leading to neglect in a system that was set up to care for such vulnerable children.

One of us took part in a consultation to a children's home in an inner-London borough. It shows the determination of a vulnerable girl to be with those who want to exploit her, and the mirroring of the inadequacy of responses and resources to help her. Interestingly these responses took the shape of a re-enactment of the initial dynamics.

The consultation took place on a fortnightly basis with the consultant spending an afternoon with the staff. At first staff failed to attend or arrived late. The pre-dominantly agency-staffed group was constantly changing and there was a high degree of permanent staff turnover. Each meeting was like starting new. It seemed impossible for them to hold in mind that there would be a consultation. They had lost three managers in quick succession and the current one was uncertain of her employment. She tried to establish the regularity of the meetings by providing lunch, but was herself often called away. In this situation it is clear that the staff would struggle to provide boundaries and consistency for young people from chaotic homes or even have a coherent perspective or model of working. Staff found it difficult to remember detailed information about young people's home backgrounds or previous experiences, despite a preoccupation with keeping adequate records and 'filling in the daily log'.

In my role as consultant they appeared to relate to me either in a deni-gratory fashion as someone who could not possibly be able to understand their situation (*'therapists don't work in the real world'* – forgetting that I was a social worker!) or with an over-idealized expectation that I would give them the answers and cure the young people. The idea that I would continue to return and remember what they had talked about the previous time seemed impossible for them to believe.

For a period of time one young woman, Amy, was brought up for discussion each week. Although the consultant had suggested initially alternating residents they presented, it was clear that Amy was in the forefront of everyone's mind, and it was realistic to spend time concentrating on her. Staff found it difficult to allow time to be interested in any links with Amy's history, as she constantly posed them with the difficulties of risk management which grabbed priority for their attention.

Amy had come into care when she was aged thirteen. Her mother died of an overdose when she was eight. Amy was looked after by a widowed grandfather whose wife had struggled throughout her life with an alcohol addiction. A series of local authority social workers had raised concerns about the quality of the grandfather's care, only to leave, and be replaced by a new social worker who 'needed time to get to know the family'. There were social services file notes describing a caring, but inadequate man, while in different entries detailing what sounded like a prurient interest in Amy's menstruation and sexual development. No one seems to have considered whether Amy's grandfather's 'intrusions' went further, and no safeguarding assessments were conducted. Amy saw herself as the 'lady of the house', and was proud of her ability to cook and clean. The grandfather saw her as 'just like her mother' but felt he could not manage without her. Yet by thirteen, Amy was deemed beyond her grandfather's control. She was staying out late, and described as being on the periphery of gang violence and drug and alcohol use. Despite her grandfather's protest, Amy came into care.

What do we know about Amy? She has lost her mother abruptly when she was eight. Her grandfather seems to have confused care and sexuality. No one had considered whether he might also have had a mild learning difficulty, although we are told that Amy was identified as having special educational needs. These learning difficulties may have contributed to why the educational aspects as well as the social aspects of school may have been problematic for her. But school staff saw her as 'high risk' and 'provocative'.

The residential care staff described during a consultation that Amy would frequently be in the sitting room in the evenings with staff, sometimes scantily dressed and sometimes in fluffy dressing gowns carrying a stuffed bear. The staff seemed perplexed by the two distinct presentations. This suggested Amy had a confused sense of herself. Her social worker and the staff were concerned that she was meeting older men (like her grandfather?), and she would often come back to the unit with cigarettes and new clothes. She would mention new 'boyfriends' who bought her jewellery. Sometimes she would return to the unit drunk and unkempt. She had started to ask her keyworker Diane about babies and if 'worms' could live in your stomach and make you sick. She denied having sex, although the 'worms' might be a confused idea of sperm. She was offered birth control and sexual health advice. A pregnancy test proved negative.

On a common-sense level Amy is lonely. She spends a lot of time in the living room near staff members. Staff were present but unable to address directly or notice properly what might be going on. Her school attendance had deteriorated and she was finding it difficult to make friends at school. The staff worried that some of the young men in the unit could 'take advantage' of her.

Like many young people in the care system a comprehensive early history is not clear. However, if her mother took an overdose when Amy was eight, it is likely that there were problems in their relationship before that. Amy seems to be sending out messages via her clothes that sometimes she is a baby wanting to be cuddled and sometimes she is a sexual person. There is confusion between sensuality and sexuality, and over generational boundaries. She may have felt that sex is the only route to physical contact or even to relationships.

What could be done to help Amy? Staff were very aware of the risks she was running and were working hard at not turning a blind eye, unlike in many sexual exploitation cases. It was decided that someone should be with Amy whenever she went out. As with many care plans it was *unrealistic*. It was also an example of how the care plan took a very concrete approach. The desire was to keep a constant eye on Amy to keep her out of harm; like a mother of a tiny baby keeping a watchful eye. However, rather than understanding that what was needed was to provide a 'symbolic eye' on Amy – in other words to offer a containing experience – the intervention was to actually be physically with her wherever she went. In this case, they asked the key worker, an attractive young black male staff member, to accompany, or at least follow Amy when she went out.

Yet what we know of Amy is that she would not experience this as concern. Instead, she soon shook him off by screaming in the street and on the bus that he is following her. Passers-by stare and attempt to intervene, and the young worker is left feeling, as he said in the consultation, 'like I am the pervert'. The watchful eye was transformed into the intrusive eye, like that of her grandfather. In telling me about it, the young worker became anxious and defensive, and the team began to express sympathy for him as the victim, generating a wave of annoyed and angry feelings at Amy and her lack of gratitude.

This is an excellent example of projective processes, and how the care becomes perverted, thus mirroring something of the earlier family dynamics and the sexual exploitation itself. It was only with opportunity to reflect and to understand these complex dynamics that the children's home continued to work with Amy and prevent a further placement breakdown, or an extended period of Amy being on the run and further at risk. In a few cases, young women like Amy are placed in secure units. However this is likely to be only a temporary measure. The main thing which will protect sexually exploited girls is a change in their way of thinking. This is of course much easier said than done when the sexual exploitation is part of a psychological defence.

A nun who rescued Nigerian women from streetwalking in Italy said 'it took a network to put them there and they need a network to get them out'. A network for Amy would include her school, the care home, her social worker and social care colleagues, and health professionals, both generic and specialist. CAMHS input would also be fundamental in working with these dynamics – although it is highly unlikely that Amy or young people like her would agree to attend therapy sessions unless the exploitation has stopped. The care network has to become, at the outset, a kind of pre-therapy therapeutic intervention. Part of the network's role is to help Amy make a space in her mind that does not rely on the omnipotent parts of her personality offering 'protection' to vulnerable parts as described above, instead coming to rely on the care provided through the network. This depends on professionals and professional groups avoiding being pulled into the familiar sado-masochistic dynamics.

Ideally, Amy should have individual psychotherapy. There is good research evidence that this helps with sexually abused girls (Long et al., 2005). Amy needs to be helped to find figures *in her mind* who are genuinely good and reliable.

Conclusion

Throughout the consultation there was an atmosphere in the home of things happening beneath the surface. One week, a very large TV was stolen '*right out from under our noses!*' When the consultant arrived one week she had noticed its absence and asked about it. Apparently one of the residents, whom I will call Chris, had during the preceding week, day-by-day and bit-by-bit, been unscrewing it from the wall bracket. The night before, a 'polite' young man had visited Chris and was introduced as a friend. He was allowed to enter and wait in the living room. While the residential worker at Chris's behest went to the kitchen to make a cup of tea, the friend went out and signalled a mate who pulled up in a car. The worker knew she should not leave the visitor alone, but equally wanted to make Chris feel like this was his home, making his friends welcome. In her absence, Chris needed only one last action to unscrew it completely and lift it off the wall, handing it out through an open window. When I commented on how something so huge was taken almost in front of their eyes, one staff member replied: 'if you really saw the extent of what happened in this place you wouldn't believe it.' Another chimed in, 'you wouldn't work here'.

Outside professionals were brought in to consult to the staff at this care home, by a manager who appreciated the struggles of working with some of the most difficult adolescents in care. Without this, institutions – including the police, health institutions and social services – can take on the shape and defences of the people they work with. In fact, perhaps because of this, Amy's workers did not turn a blind eye to the risks she took although not surprisingly they still found her behaviours difficult to manage.

It is human to want to turn away from what social workers are asked to face. Keeping an eye on many disturbed and disturbing young people is a mammoth task. It needs skill and support, and a theoretical framework that helps to explain why it is so difficult to see. At a social gathering the other evening I was speaking to a woman who, when hearing I was a social worker, said she couldn't do what I do:

> You must see such awful things all the time. I couldn't do it. When I read a book and I know there is going to be something horrible happening I have to skip those pages – I can't look at them. My sister when she knows I've done it

makes a meal of telling me all of the gory details. She derides me for looking away. I guess it's a privilege not to have to see what's in front of your nose.

Afterword

Many victims of sexual exploitation are known to social workers or actually in the care system. Almost by definition they have families who have found it hard to care for them. Common reasons for this are mental health problems or drug and alcohol use. However a colleague recently told us that increasingly girls from 'ordinary' families are being targeted. They are picked up in ordinary places, such as shoe shops. How do we explain this? As a society we do not care well for more vulnerable members – the elderly, the mentally ill and, of course, children. Increasingly those who care for children, usually mothers, are pressurised to return to work. Young children are cared for in day nurseries or in a patchwork of arrangements. These arrangements can be very good or unsatisfactory. For example, research shows that group care is unhelpful for children under a year old (McGurk, 1993), yet many day nurseries offer care for children as young as three months. A vulnerable child in a difficult environment may turn to omnipotent aspects of his or her mind. They may develop an internal world that resonates with the gangs of exploiters. In the 1960s a filmmaker, James Robertson, followed the progress of a 17-month-old boy 'John', who spent nine days in a residential nursery while his mother was having a baby. Owing to the shift system, it was impossible for any child to form a consistent relationship with a member of staff. Most of the children gave up turning to an adult. Instead they formed an excited, quarrelsome gang. We believe this pattern is a precursor of the state of mind of girls or boys who are seduced by an exciting gang of exploiters. For a while residential nurseries were closed down. They are beginning to open again.

We are aware that boys as well as girls are the victims of sexual exploitation. As this book was going to press the scandal was just breaking of the abuse of young boys by charismatic football coaches. In keeping with the usual pattern of sexual abuse, the clubs and the Football Association seemed to have turned a blind eye. At the moment, not enough is known about the individual cases. However, the larger pattern of denial continues. 'It could not happen now.' There is an urgent need for research in this area. We need to understand the ingredients of effective help for victims. We also need to know what enables young people to resist these pressures. We believe it is an internal world of helpful maternal and paternal figures.

References

Basch, H. (1983) The perception of reality and the disavowal of meaning. *The Annual of Psychoanalysis* 11, 125–153.

Britton, R. (1994) The blindness of the seeing eye: inverse symmetry as a defense against reality. *Psychoanalytic Inquiry* 14(3), 365–378.

Casey, L. (2016) *The Casey Review: A Review into Opportunity and Integration.* London: UK Government.

Home Office (2015) *Tackling Child Sexual Exploitation.* Available from: www.gov.uk/governm ent/uploads/system/uploads/attachment_data/file/408604/ [accessed 6 February 2017].

Jay, A. (2014) *Independent Inquiry into Child Sexual Exploitation in Rotherham (1997–2013).* Rotherham: Rotherham Metropolitan Borough Council.

Long, J., Trowell, J. and Miles, G. (2005) Individual brief psychotherapy with sexually abused girls and parallel support work with parents and carers. In: Bower, M. (ed.) *Thinking Under Fire: Psychoanalytic Theory for Social Work Practice.* London: Routledge.

McGurk, H., Caplan, M., Henessey, E. and Moss, P. (1993) Controversy, theory and social context in contemporary day care research. *Journal of Clinical Psychology and Psychotherapy* 32(1), 3–23.

Milton, J. (1994) Abuser and abused: Perverse solutions following childhood abuse. *Psychoanalytic Psychotherapy* 8, 243–255.

Rosenfeld, H. (1971) A clinical approach to the psychoanalytic theory of the life and death instincts. *International Journal of Psychoanalysis* 52, 169–178.

Steiner, J. (1993) *Psychic Retreats.* London: Routledge.

12

GETTING THE BALANCE RIGHT

Helping young people with a learning disability achieve independence

Susan Chantrell

Introduction

Parenting, child and adolescent development, and the achievement of independence for young people are complex processes. Our usual expectation is that there will be a gradual increase in independence for young people, who will become more able to: spend time away from home; travel independently; have a social and love life; find work and support themselves financially; move out of the family home, become fully independent and possibly parents themselves. Parents can gradually get on with their own lives: they might become grandparents offering further support to their children and grandchildren; and they might need support from their own children in older age. Siblings may develop lifelong satisfying and supportive relationships with each other. Of course we all know that this is complicated with endless variations. Young people can fluctuate between seeking and achieving independence and returning to their parents' home for support along the way, and the eventual outcome can vary.

For young people with a learning disability and their parents this process can be even more complex. The young people might not be able to achieve such full independence, with varied consequences for themselves and family. As a child and adolescent psychotherapist, I have had the opportunity to meet many families dealing with these issues in different ways. I have noticed that the best situation seems to be one in which there is balance in the family between providing a safe, protecting home while at the same time allowing the young person to develop as much independent functioning as they are capable of and want to achieve, inside and beyond the home. But it can be difficult to get this balance right. Times of change and transition can be challenging, for example changing schools or as other young people in the family move on in life in a more ordinary way. There can be practical issues which get in the way, such as availability of suitable opportunities for young people with a learning disability to have an independent social life, appropriate work and housing. However there can also be complex psychological issues, for both the young people and their families, which can get in the way of getting this balance right, and it is this area which will be explored in this chapter.

I will first present some statistics concerning the mental health of children and young people with a learning disability. I will give some information about the literature on psychoanalytic psychotherapy with people with a learning disability, and introduce the concepts of 'emotional intelligence' and 'secondary handicap'. I will then discuss some of the psychological difficulties faced by parents, the children and young people, and their siblings. I will give some illustrations based on my case work; these illustrations are not of actual patients but are of situations and interactions taken into a different context and anonymised to preserve patient confidentiality.

The mental health of children and young people with a learning disability

In a study 'The Mental Health of Children and Adolescents with Learning Disabilities in Britain', Emerson and Hatton (2007) found that 36 per cent of children and adolescents, aged between 5 and 16 years, have a diagnosable 'psychiatric disorder'. 'Psychiatric disorder' includes diagnoses such as 'emotional disorder' (which covers anxiety and mood disorders), conduct disorder and ADHD (Attention Deficit and Hyperactivity Disorder). This level of diagnosable psychiatric disorder is about six times the prevalence in their non-learning disabled peers.

The picture that Emerson and Hatton discuss is made more complex by the fact that children and young people with a learning disability tend to be poorer, to suffer from more challenging life circumstances and to have fewer friends, all of which in themselves are factors which increase the risk of mental health difficulties in children. Emerson and Hatton estimated that about two-thirds of the difference in prevalence of diagnosable psychiatric disorders could be attributed to the above factors rather than to the learning disability itself. However, that leaves one-third of the risk attributable to the learning disability itself and they speculated about the contribution of intellectual impairment in 'reducing the capacity for finding creative and adaptive solutions to life's challenges'. In this chapter I will discuss the emotional difficulties for both the young people with a learning disability and their families, and will return to the issue of increased risk of mental health difficulties in my discussion.

Psychoanalytic psychotherapy with people with a learning disability

I sometimes encounter the view, expressed by professionals, that people with a learning disability cannot benefit from psychotherapy, because it requires a 'normal' or higher than average cognitive ability. However, this is not the case. There are many accounts of psychoanalytic psychotherapy and psychoanalytically informed work with learning disabled children, adolescents, adults, their families and professionals working with them (Hodges, 2003; Sinason, 2010; Stokes, 1987; Simpson et al., 2004; Symington, 1981). There is possibly an image of psychoanalytic psychotherapists practising only the 'talking cure'. However, the 'talking cure' also involves close observation and attention to non-verbal communications and the countertransference, in addition to what is said. Sinason (2010) suggests that Child and Adolescent Psychotherapists are particularly well-suited to working with learning disabled patients, because we are so used to working with patients of different ages and developmental levels, who communicate in such a variety of ways, such as through play and drawing.

In his paper 'Insights from psychotherapy', Jon Stokes (1987) wrote that it was useful to distinguish between 'emotional intelligence' and 'cognitive intelligence'. Emotional intelligence is the capacity to be in touch with and express feelings. He pointed out that there is no clear one-to-one relationship between emotional and cognitive intelligence. Someone who scores low in a cognitive intelligence test can be highly emotionally intelligent. Conversely, a person can be cognitively highly intelligent but lacking in emotional intelligence.

Stokes (1987), Sinason (2010) and others have written about 'secondary handicap' or 'secondary handicapping processes'. If the actual, organic 'handicap' is 'primary', the defensive use or exaggeration of it is the 'secondary handicap'. We all have to come to terms with our limitations, e.g. that we will not be as successful as we might have hoped to be. However, Sinason points out how much more difficult and painful this is if your limitations are 'concretely defined by brain damage or chromosomal abnormality' and possibly visible to all. Powerful defences are mobilised against this pain, including secondary handicapping processes. For example, a learning disabled person might act as more learning disabled than they actually are, which can serve various functions. One is that, if there is an omnipotent phantasy that the disability can be controlled through exaggeration, there can also be a phantasy that it could be removed altogether. Or it might be easier to be seen as someone more severely disabled and avoid real contact with others, who might too clearly perceive the painful reality of one's actual, if lesser, limitations.

The concepts of 'emotional intelligence' and 'secondary handicap' have relevance to us all. Jon Stokes (1987) gives the example of an adolescent who, in the face of not doing very well in exams, might say 'I only failed because I didn't work hard enough', which is easier than saying 'I brought failure on myself because I came up against something I could not manage'. In psychotherapy treatment we are essentially attempting to increase emotional intelligence and lessen secondary handicapping processes.

In this chapter I will not be concentrating on the important areas of sexuality and cultural differences. For more consideration of these areas, I recommend Sinason (2010) and Usiskin (2004).

Difficulties faced by children and young people with a learning disability and their families

When a baby is born into a family, the parents will inevitably have their fantasies, both conscious and unconscious, about what the baby and growing child will be like. Will the child be a boy or girl, what will he or she look like, what sort of character and talents will they have, will they get along well with their parents and siblings? In all families there is an adjustment when the real baby arrives and develops. Some things about him or her might accord with the fantasy or might conflict in both positive and negative ways. To an extent all parents have to 'mourn' the loss of the fantasised child.

However, a baby might be born with an identifiable disability. It might become apparent as time goes on that there is a disability or something might happen during development, e.g. an illness or accident, which causes a disability. In different ways, these situations even more strongly involve the loss of the hoped for, fantasised child. Some writers, for example Simpson (2005), have referred to the 'narcissistic injury' or 'wound' experienced by parents in these circumstances. How have they managed to produce a disabled child? They might feel it is their fault in some way, even if told the opposite by professionals, with resulting feelings of guilt and shame. Child psychotherapist Shirley Hoxter (1986), writing about her work with physically disabled patients, has discussed the traumatic aspect of the discovery of disability. Hoxter suggested that each re-encounter with and acknowledgement of the disability also has a traumatic dimension.

In Melanie Klein's model of human development, we each face a lifelong struggle to integrate our feelings of love and hate, to achieve a balance between conflicting feelings for the same other person or object. Parents of a child with a disability face additional challenges. The fantasised perfect baby is actually disabled and this provokes a potent mixture of loving and protective feelings, but also of anger, grief, pain, anxiety, guilt and shame. There might also be hatred or disgust, which are very hard to experience and have to be strongly defended against psychologically. All parents are individuals and some find a disabled child more difficult to deal with, perhaps depending on the nature of their own life experiences and inner world.

Instead of the child who will develop in the usual way, moving gradually towards independence, parents of a child with a learning disability face a different path. This can include seeking and digesting diagnoses, and possibly what can feel like a lifetime of appointments and struggles to access appropriate resources. Parents with their own life and career aspirations might lose some of those possibilities and face an alternative 'career' as the carers and advocates for their disabled child.

How can parents cope with the complicated and painful situation outlined above? In a parental couple there might be a fantasy that the other is somehow to blame, has caused the difficulty. Not infrequently I have come across a situation where one parent seems less worried and the other very worried and preoccupied; there seems to be a split between their attitudes. This might be accompanied by an idea that the less worried parent has 'come to terms' with the difficulty and does not need to talk about it. There might even be a denial in one parent that the difficulty really exists, and an idea that the other parent, through his or her worry, has sought a diagnosis and got it. The other parent is then the one who is 'overly anxious', 'over-involved', making things worse. The couple are then not able to turn to each other for the support and containment they need. In work with parents we sometimes notice this and have to work carefully and tactfully to help. Some parents are single parents with the added burden this involves; Emerson and Hatton (2007) reported that 30 per cent of the children and young people in their study were supported by a single parent. Simpson (2005) draws attention to depression in parents of children with a learning disability and a high level of deterioration in the marital relationship or break up.

The early years of infancy and young childhood are vital in the emotional development of a child. In healthy emotional development a child is cared for by a parent or parents who are not too stressed and are able to provide an emotionally receptive environment in which the infant's feelings can be thoughtfully and consistently contained. In this sort of environment the infant/young child develops the capacity to contain their own emotions, of both love and hate, and to achieve a firm sense of a good internal object in a predominantly benign rather than persecutory inner world. With these emotional achievements comes the capacity to make and sustain satisfying personal relationships, to have an interest in the external world and to learn. But how is this affected when the parent(s) are struggling with the emotions outlined above? I have discussed the psychological situation for parents first, because this is the crucible in which the early stages of emotional development take place and will inevitably affect that process. For a very full discussion of the emotional problems facing parents of children with a learning disability, see Simpson (2005).

As the growing child increasingly comes into contact with the world outside the family, there are additional challenges. There is the pain and humiliation of difference, which might depend on how apparent the disability is and how it is perceived in society. There are also the additional difficulties with becoming independent in the usual way, of making friends and developing an independent social life, of sexuality, of gaining meaningful work, financial independence and leaving home. The usual adolescent struggles are further complicated. There may also be a painful comparison with siblings and peers, who are more able to progress in life. How to deal with anger, envy, sadness, shame and frustration when dependent?

Parents may deal with their painful feelings about their child by using defences of denial or idealisation, for example: by denying that the child is aware of their difference; by idealising the child as not having negative or sexual thoughts and feelings; and by not linking the child's emotional and behavioural presentation with their thoughts and feelings.

While we all do have different temperaments and some children and young people may be more or less equable, it is highly unlikely that anyone, disabled or otherwise, does not have negative feelings. A consequence of this sort of view is that there is sometimes a failure to link emotional or behavioural difficulties to negative feelings, because it is too difficult to bear that children and young people with a learning disability have such feelings. Children and young people with a learning disability who cannot express their emotions or feel that any negative emotions are unwelcome can develop challenging behaviour, become depressed or anxious, or suffer emotional breakdown.

I have previously written (Chantrell, 2009) about a little girl who I saw in weekly psychotherapy from age eight to eleven, while a colleague saw her parents together for monthly sessions. Ellie had a global developmental delay and a mild learning disability (IQ in range 55–69) and was referred because of her rough and erratic behaviour at her special school. The school initially thought that her rough behaviour had no meaning or understandable trigger. But when Ellie was helped to develop in her emotional intelligence, able to better identify her feelings and begin to express them in words, her rough behaviour subsided.

While it can be difficult for a parent to be in touch with all their mixed feelings about their disabled child, it is additionally painful to know that the child might be aware of their difference and have their own feelings about it. For example, Ellie's parents thought she was not aware of her difference, especially since she attended a special school. They thought it best to preserve her innocent state of not knowing and feared that it would be cruel to do the opposite. However, from the content of her sessions, I thought that Ellie was aware of her difference and sometimes felt sad and humiliated. There would often be times in sessions when Ellie could not do something competently, such as putting the lid on a toy baby bottle, and felt angry, upset and frustrated with her efforts. She would then say 'can't do it' or express that something was 'broken'. Sometimes she put the rubbish bin on her head, which seemed an eloquent non-verbal communication. When the subject was discussed with her parents in a review meeting, they suddenly remembered that when she was aged six, Ellie had been playing with a group of younger children. Ellie had remarked that she was bigger than the others, in a way that her parents thought indicated that she had an idea that she was the same age as the others but just bigger.

Thinking that their child realises and is angry, sad or ashamed about their difference is very hard for parents to bear and they can feel that it is cruel to acknowledge it. However, lack of acknowledgement might feed into the child's own need to deny the painful reality of their disability. Even worse, the child might come to feel that it is a shameful subject, something that cannot be acknowledged or discussed. Hoxter (1986), thinking about physically disabled patients, discusses co-existing states of knowing and unknowing. She writes

> When working with the physically disabled it is essential that the therapist should not collude with a denial of the disability. It is equally essential that re-encounters with the traumatic should not be thrust upon the patient like a surgical instrument. Sensitive modulation may be required to enable the repetitions of the trauma to lead towards integration rather than to further repetitions of splitting and repression – or overwhelming despair.
>
> *(Hoxter, 1986: 95)*

For siblings, the emotional situation of having a learning disabled sibling is also complex. The place of a normally developing sibling, to be friends with and/or argue with, is occupied by a disabled brother or sister, and this might also be experienced as a loss and provoke difficult mixed feelings. Their parents are affected and their attention may be drawn away to the more vulnerable disabled child. Siblings might unconsciously fear that they have caused the damage, for example if the disabled child is younger and the older sibling felt supplanted by the new brother or sister. Siblings might think or fear that they will be responsible for their disabled sibling when the parents get older or die. Some siblings might become interested in the field of disability and embark on a career in the caring professions. There are others who struggle with more negative feelings. And in a family with more than one sibling, there might be different attitudes amongst them.

In one family I worked with, there was a learning disabled sister aged twelve and a younger brother aged ten. The parents reported that their son's teacher had told them that he was very kind to disabled or vulnerable children at school. However there was a lot of conflict between the siblings at home, and his parents had felt upset when their son said to them that he wished his sister was not learning disabled. This was painful for the parents to hear, partly because it accorded with their own mixed feelings about their daughter's disability, which they were also struggling with.

Each family develops its own way of coping with these complex feelings and these ways of coping might promote or inhibit the emotional development of the young person with a learning disability and other family members. As stated earlier, I have noticed that the best situation seems to be one in which there is balance in the family between providing a safe, protecting home while at the same time allowing the young person to develop as much independent functioning as they are capable of and want to achieve, inside and beyond the home.

A good example of getting the balance right was John, who I first met in a clinic I worked in when he was aged 16. John was from a white, not well-off family and had a mild learning disability. He had extra help at his secondary school and he had been badly bullied there. His mother was concerned about the coming transition to college including that he could not travel independently on a bus. There was an initial idea in the clinic that John might benefit from individual psychotherapy. However the clinician who assessed him found that John would not separate from his mother to have time alone with her. So it was agreed that I would offer John and his mother monthly sessions together. I got to know that John lived with his single mother and an older sister. They lived in cramped conditions in a two-bedroom property, where mother slept in the living room so that her two children could have their own private spaces. John's mother impressed me as someone who very appropriately supported and advocated for her son. For example, she persisted in trying various ways of helping him to travel to school on the bus, she encouraged him to go out on his own to the local shops to buy things he liked, or to go to the cinema with a friend. He developed a strong friendship with another learning disabled young man who liked similar things and they could visit each other in their respective family homes. John's friend liked to travel around on trains, visiting particular landmarks related to his special interest, and John happily joined him in this. It was clear from some of his accounts of these trips that John and his friend were sometimes bullied by youths but they managed to weather this together. Gradually John began to travel on his own on buses. Overall I thought that John's mother helped him, in a gentle but persistent way, to develop what independence was possible for him, while recognising his limitations and making space for him in her home. When her daughter moved out to live with a partner, John's mother had her own bedroom again after many years of patient waiting. John's mother did not work outside the home and did not express a desire to do so, and this was probably a factor which was helpful.

In contrast, I have come across other family situations in which young people, as able as John, might be constantly accompanied and cared for, and not encouraged to go out on their own or to develop independent functioning. In John's family, since his mother did not work outside the home or travel away from home, it was perhaps easier to provide a simple and consistent lifestyle based around the family home and locality. In families where a parent or both parents are pursuing their own careers, this can add extra pressures on the family as well as the benefits in terms of the mental wellbeing of the working parent and family finances.

For example, Angela was a young adult with a moderate learning disability (IQ in range 40–55) who was referred for weekly psychotherapy. Angela had effectively suffered a mental breakdown which seemed associated with changes in her family as her older siblings moved on in life. Angela's was a Western European family, and her parents were successful and busy academics who had been settled in the UK for many years and their children had been born here. Angela had an older brother and sister, who had both completed their university degrees and were developing their careers and relationships. There was someone with or looking out for Angela at all times and she seemed to lack any drive to become more independent. Her family lived a busy and creative lifestyle, with many contacts with extended family and friends, cultural events and trips abroad. So on the surface Angela had an active and interesting life, and yet she had become unwell. Her parents were understandably worried about what the future might hold for her. As I heard more about her life in the sessions, I began to feel that she was living in the shadows of her well-meaning family. I began to wonder if she would prosper better in a more ordinary set-up, such as John's, in which she could have a more predictable, if duller, life from which she could gradually develop more independence. I will discuss some aspects of Angela's psychotherapy later in this chapter.

Helping children and young people with a learning disability with their feelings

I have set out some of the emotional difficulties which I believe are faced by children and young people with learning disabilities and their families. I would now like to discuss some ways in which professionals might become receptive to the feelings of the children and young people they work with, so that they can be more effective in helping them and their families.

As a psychoanalytic child and adolescent psychotherapist, I start from the point of view that all behaviour is potentially meaningful. This means that I attend to verbal communication but also to non-verbal communication, which includes general behaviour, play, drawing, the role I seem to be assigned by patients and the feelings evoked in me by being with them. I have been trained to observe my patients and my own emotional states, to think in terms of unconscious processes, transference, countertransference, projection and container/contained relationships. This helps me to be aware of what is being communicated to me, both verbally and non-verbally, and also if there might seem to be inhibitions in communicating certain feelings and ideas.

I will give some examples of different kinds of communications with patients and how I have understood them. I hope this will be helpful to other professionals who might gain confidence to listen to and observe their clients' communications including the emotional effect they have on them. It is not necessary to be seeing patients in a therapeutic setting to expand awareness in this respect and apply psychoanalytic theory.

With John and his mother, we talked. I saw them over a period of more than two years. At first John's mother did most of the talking about John and their family life. As John got used to the sessions, a pattern developed in which his mother would talk for part of the session and then John would bring in his own thoughts. For example John's mother was separated from his father and she started a relationship with a man called Dave, who began to stay overnight and eventually moved in with them. John began to complain about Dave in the sessions. He objected to having to share the television in the living room with Dave and disliked that Dave had seemed to assume some authority over him. This in turn helped John to talk about his wish that his mother and father would get back together. John's mother indicated to me that it was a new development for John to talk about things like this; she had not known his feelings but had been aware of some difficult atmospheres and behaviour at home. It took time for John to be able to talk like this and it set in train a helpful process, in which John and his mother were able to talk about important things together. It seemed that both were increasing in emotional intelligence. For example his mother helped John to see that, while he had his own bedroom, she and Dave only had the living room and so this was difficult for them too. I think that when John started to be able to express his feelings, positive and negative, about all manner of subjects over the course of time, this helped the family to live together successfully and for John to feel more confident and able to grow in independence. After his treatment had ended I met John by chance at a bus station. He got onto the bus I was taking, making it clear that he had a choice of buses he could take but was choosing this one. He had a friend with him and he introduced me as the woman he used to see at the clinic and who had helped him. He even seemed to imply that his friend could benefit from similar help. Apart from the positive feedback, it was also pleasing to see him travelling around so confidently.

John was very keen on films about super heroes who had 'special powers' or were 'mutants' and he would often explain the plots to me. I thought that this interest partly related to his feelings about being different, a desire to be able to change, and to be different in a good or superior way. I think it is always useful to think about the stories that are interesting to young people, in films or books, and what the plot-lines might mean to them. Stories such as *Star Wars* are our modern-day fairy tales. Fairy tales include lovely princesses and horrible witches, and ideas of transformation from a 'frog' into someone good and beautiful. But Sinason (1999: 197), writing about disabled adolescents struggling with the problem of their difference, writes: 'And it does not go away. They are not going to be the frog that turns into a prince; they are going to stay the frog.' Maybe the transformative aspect of these stories carries a particular meaning for disabled children and young people.

In another example, I was at a social services office and included in a discussion about a young man with a learning disability. He had been causing a lot of difficulty at a respite care facility he had recently started to attend by repeatedly trying to set off the fire alarm. It seemed that this was seen as challenging behaviour and the staff were at a loss as to how to deal with it. In the discussion it was suggested that his behaviour might be a habit and that he got attention when he did it. However, we also wondered if he might be very anxious or afraid in the respite care, worried about his family or that he might not be able to return home, and that his wanting to call the fire brigade might be meaningful.

Another more disturbing case was of Mary, aged 16. Mary had cerebral palsy and a mild learning disability. Mary could walk but was visibly disabled and spoke in a slurred voice. Social Services and Mary's school had been concerned for some time about Mary's care by her single mother, who seemed unsupportive and sometimes punitive. Mary was popular with the staff at her school where she adopted a rather cheeky persona, always laughing and joking with the special needs staff. But they noted that she seemed reluctant to go home and did not look forward to the school holidays. A colleague was working with Mary's mother, school and social worker, and asked me to see Mary on her own. I saw Mary weekly for a few months. She was brought to her sessions by a favourite learning assistant, Pat. When I collected Mary from the waiting room, she would be engaged in cheeky banter with Pat, telling her to 'behave yourself' and to go out and get her some crisps or a fizzy drink.

As we took the lift up to my room there would be a marked change in Mary, as if she shed the cheeky persona and let me see the Mary it covered. In the first session Mary found the toy mirror in the dolls' house, looked into it and cried 'I'm ugly'. This was not repeated. I thought that Mary's behaviour in the waiting room was like a 'secondary handicap'; she actually drew more attention to herself and seemed more disabled than she was, but this covered the real disabled girl underneath who was sad and feared that she was 'ugly'.

Also in the first session Mary told me that she would talk to me about her mother. Verbally, she did not. However, she proceeded to play with a teddy in a way that continued over the sessions. In my room I had a toy cradle filled with cuddly toys, cups and saucers, phone and medical kit. Mary would play that the teddy was a baby who was not well, crying and being sick. Mary played the baby's mother or sometimes she wanted me to play that role. When Mary was the mother, she complained that the baby had made her clothes dirty by being sick on her, was naughty and sometimes she hit the baby. When I was the mother, Mary wanted me to do the same as she did. However, I spoke to the baby in a different way and asked what was the matter and suggested that the baby could not help being sick. While Mary listened, she also made it clear that the baby was being naughty sometimes and that I should not be fooled. In the play the doctor would be called and, playing this role, I would carefully examine the baby and talk to the mother (Mary) about it.

I thought that Mary was powerfully communicating to me about the care she was used to with her own mother. She was 'talking to me about her mother' but through play. She was also communicating to me that she had become a not entirely passive partner in her relationship with her mother. In the transference, I was the doctor she was bringing her baby self to see. It is interesting that Mary was sixteen, but she was able to play with toys and show me her thoughts and feelings in this way. It could seem patronising to offer toys to an adolescent, but since I also saw children, I just had these in my therapy room. If not working in a room with toys, I would routinely make drawing and some craft materials available to an adolescent, in case they want to use them. I did not see Mary for long, as it became difficult for her school to bring her. However, my colleague carried on working with her family and we thought that issues concerning Mary's care were of most importance. Interestingly, I heard sometime later that Mary had developed an illness and was admitted to hospital. No physical cause was found for the illness. The hospital tried to discharge her but she refused to give up the idea that she was unwell and could not return home.

I would like to return to my patient Angela now, who I saw weekly for two years while her parents were seen at intervals by a colleague. From the outset Angela seemed accepting of the weekly arrangement to see me. She was always brought to the sessions by a family member or helper. She seemed quite passive and often referred to people she knew as a 'nice woman' or the like. I felt that I might become another 'nice woman' who she came to see, another member of the system in which she was always with someone else. Early on in her therapy, in a session she looked at her watch and I suggested that maybe she was a bit 'fed-up' with coming here and that the session might seem too long. Although Angela did not express agreement, she continued to sometimes pointedly look at her watch in sessions and smile, I thought rather mischievously, and I made a similar interpretation. I began to feel that it was important to notice and encourage Angela to express her more negative feelings, considering that this might help her to develop her emotional intelligence and a stronger sense of her own desires and wishes.

Over time there were other examples of Angela starting to express more of her negative feelings to me. I had been wearing skirts and shirts to our sessions, thinking that I looked smart and professional. However, one day I had possibly ended up looking rather like a policewoman, in a navy blue skirt and striped shirt.

Angela looked me up and down and asked if I was wearing a man's shirt, with an amused look on her face. I suggested that she did not think much to my look today, that I did not look quite right. On another occasion she had been brought to her session by a female helper, who I assumed was another of her female helpers and so called her by the wrong name. Angela observed this and would often return to it in sessions, remembering the day when I had got something wrong which she thought had been highly embarrassing. In these examples Angela projected into me her own feelings of not looking quite right or getting things wrong. I thought this was positive and encouraged her to say these things. I think she was possibly also expressing her envy of me as a non-learning disabled person.

In another session Angela told me that there had been a box of chocolates at home. The chocolates were a kind she particularly liked and she had taken them off to her room to eat them. Her sister had been looking for them, had called Angela but she had not answered and this had caused an argument. I suggested that she had thought something like – 'I like these yummy chocolates and I want to eat them all up and no one else is going to have one!' Angela looked amused and asked me to 'say that again'. I thought it important to notice and validate her greed.

Over time Angela became more able to assert herself in small ways in her family. For example, she was able to say that she did not want to do something with her family that would mean missing another activity she wanted to do. Reporting on a family weekend away, she was able to express that she wished someone had talked with her more. Although, while I was seeing her, Angela did not develop much more actual independence, I thought these were small but positive signs of progress.

Lastly I would like to discuss the danger of being incorporated into a family's way of operating and replicating it. I had been seeing a young man called Paul, aged nineteen, for weekly psychotherapy for some time. Paul had a mild learning disability and was, like Angela, in a family where he was not developing much independence. I saw him in a clinic which had a Child and Family, Adolescent and Adult Departments which were on different floors with different waiting rooms. My team was an all-age team but I usually used rooms in the Child and Family Department. I had been seeing Paul in a room in the Child and Family Department, which meant that he and his parents would come to the waiting room and be surrounded by children. His parents were also seen monthly by a colleague, who collected them from the Child and Family waiting room. After discussion in the team, it was decided that I should start seeing Paul in the Adolescent Department, which was more age appropriate. We decided that my colleague would continue to collect his parents from the Child and Family Department which meant that sometimes Paul would have to come up to the Adolescent Department on his own, announce that he had arrived and wait for me.

At first Paul found this change disconcerting and he would say that he missed the Child and Family waiting room. I found myself feeling anxious that he might somehow get lost finding his way up to the Adolescent Department without his parents, but he did not.

The next challenge was that, after sessions, I walked him back to the Adolescent Department waiting room and sometimes left him there to wait for his parents. I was again aware of feeling anxious, this time that he might wander off and not meet up with his parents, but this did not happen.

I then realised that I could let him walk back down a set of stairs and along a corridor from my room to the Adolescent Department waiting room. At first he used to come back to my room after a couple of minutes and look in to check that I was still there. But he managed to find his way back to the waiting room. Over time he still said he missed the Child and Family Department but he also began to wonder when he might go up to the Adult Department.

In Paul's case I felt anxious that he would get lost in the gaps between rooms without someone looking out for him. It felt important to feel this, as if it gave me a small taste of what it must have been like for his parents. As professionals we might encourage parents to promote the independence of their learning disabled young people but it is perhaps hard to truly appreciate the strength of the anxiety parents feel.

Sometimes, parents' unconscious negative feelings towards the child or young person might paradoxically make it more difficult to allow the child to separate. If a parent unconsciously wishes that their child was not there, it might seem too anxiety-provoking to create the situation in which this could become a reality.

Discussion

I have suggested that for a young person with a learning disability, the best situation seems to be one in which there is balance in the family between providing a safe, protecting home while at the same time allowing the young person to develop as much independent functioning as they are capable of and want to achieve, inside and beyond the home. But it can be difficult to get this balance right. I have discussed some of the psychological issues that complicate this, for the young person, parents and other family members. As well as the positives in family life, there are negative and painful feelings which can get in the way. Psychological defences are necessary but can also be unhelpful. Sometimes the family can seem to be functioning well but then something can cause things to go out of balance again, e.g. when young people have to change school.

Emerson and Hatton (2007) estimated that about two-thirds of the difference in prevalence of diagnosable psychiatric disorders, between learning disabled young people and their peers, could be attributed to factors other than to the learning disability itself. They included relative poverty, suffering from more challenging life circumstances and having fewer friends, all of which are factors that increase the risk of mental health difficulties in children and young people. In addition to the organic difficulty, I think that the complex family and individual psychological situation accounts for the other third of the risk. The learning disabled child is born into a potentially difficult set of circumstances in which parents are traumatised, grieving, with conflicting emotions and a damaged capacity for reverie and containment. It is not surprising that the ordinary emotional achievements, which are the basis of good mental health, are compromised. By the ordinary emotional achievements, I mean the capacity to contain one's own emotions, of both love and hate, and to achieve a firm sense of a good internal object in a pre-dominantly benign rather than persecutory inner world. With these emotional achievements comes the capacity to make and sustain satisfying personal relation-ships, to have an interest in the external world and to learn.

Factors in the external world are also of vital importance. Ready access to social activities where friendships can be made is so important for mental health. I thought that it made such a positive difference to my patient, John, when he found a good friend. Having his friend encouraged John to gain more independence, gave him pleasure and prevented him from being lonely. In contrast my patient Angela found it difficult to spend much time with other similar young people, amongst whom she might have found a friend. Transport, work opportunities and housing are also very important. Unfortunately all of these things are less available in the age of austerity and cut-backs.

The social worker has a role which includes understanding the psychological diffi-culties of her clients and their families and helping them to access helpful services such as social activities, transport, work and housing. I hope that this chapter will contribute to helping social workers with their clients, by being confident to use their own 'therapeutic' capacities to observe, notice their own emotional responses, listen and build helping relationships. If social workers consider that additional psychological help is needed for their clients, they can refer for psychotherapy or counselling if there are suitable services available. Support for parents is of course very important.

Editors' afterword

This chapter provides a very comprehensive view of some of the developmental issues for learning disabled children and their parents. It makes it clear that many learning disabled people may have greater awareness of their difficulties than they are sometimes credited with.

Work with learning disabled people can raise difficult ethical issues, particularly when they become parents. One of us worked with a single learning disabled woman who had a nine-year-old daughter of normal intelligence. They came to the attention of social services because the neighbours complained about the smell of their flat. Miss A had left home to become the 'housekeeper' of an elderly man who was Jennifer's father. He had subsequently died. From an early age Jennifer was in effect her mother's carer. The bond between them was strong, but Jennifer had no friends or social life. For example, Jennifer had to do all the shopping because Ms A could not manage money. At the time of the referral there was a precarious equilibrium between mother and daughter, however things would probably become more precarious as Jennifer entered adolescence.

Learning disability often has a genetic basis. However Valerie Sinason (1999, 2010) has described a sort of learning disability which is acquired, usually through trauma – particularly sexual abuse. In this situation the child dissociates themselves from awareness, often as a means of psychic survival. Massive neglect can also have a similar effect. It is not usually enough to place the child in a more ordinary environment. There has to be an opportunity to work through previous experiences. It is well known that children in the care system often do badly at school. The reasons for this are often complex, but must often be an emotionally related learning disability. Unfortunately the supply of educational psychologists and child psychotherapists is limited. As is often the case, the social worker looks round for a resource and finds that they are 'it'. Awareness of these issues can still helpfully inform work with these young people.

References

Chantrell, S. (2009) Growth in emotional intelligence. Psychotherapy with a learning disabled girl. *Journal of Child Psychotherapy* 35(2), 157–174.

Emerson, E. and Hatton, C. (2007) *The Mental Health of Children and Adolescents with Learning Disabilities in Britain*. Lancaster: Institute for Health Research, Lancaster University.

Hodges, S. (2003) *Counselling Adults with Learning Disabilities*. Basingstoke: Palgrave, Macmillan.

Hoxter, S. (1986) The significance of trauma in the difficulties encountered by physically disabled children. *Journal of Child Psychotherapy* 12(1), 87–103.

Simpson, D. (2005) Psychoanalytic perspectives on emotional problems facing parents of children with learning disabilities. In: Bower, M. (ed.) *Psychoanalytic Theory for Social Work Practice. Thinking under Fire*. London: Routledge, pp. 103–111.

Simpson, D. and Miller, L. (eds) (2004) *Unexpected Gains: Psychotherapy with People with Learning Disabilities*. London: Karnac.

Sinason, V. (1999) Psychoanalysis and mental handicap: experience from the Tavistock Clinic. In: De Groef, J. and Heinemann, E. (eds) *Psychoanalysis and Mental Handicap*. London: Free Association Books.

Sinason, V. (2010) *Mental Handicap and the Human Condition. An Analytic Approach to Intellectual Disability*, 2nd edn. London: Free Association Books.

Stokes, J. (1987) Insights from Psychotherapy. Paper presented at International Symposium on Mental Handicap, Royal Society of Medicine, 25 February.

Symington, N. (1981) The psychotherapy of a subnormal patient. *British Journal Medical Psychology* 54, 187–199.

Usiskin, J. (2004) Some thoughts on psychotherapeutic work with learning-disabled children and their parents from orthodox religious communities. In: Simpson, D. and Miller, L. (eds) *Unexpected Gains: Psychotherapy with People with Learning Disabilities*, 1st edn. London: Karnac.

13

WORKING WITH TRAUMATISED REFUGEES

Joanne Stubley

A refugee in Britain is someone who has obtained refuge under the terms of the 1951 United Nations convention relating to the status of refugees, which defines refugees as

> people who, because of a well-founded fear of persecution, for reasons of race, religion, nationality, membership of a particular social group or political opinion, leave their country of origin and are unable or unwilling to avail themselves of the protection of that country.

A refugee may well have faced multiple bereavements including loss of country, status, activity, cultural reference points, social networks and family. They may have faced persistent and intensive persecution, witnessed violence inflicted on loved ones or had violence senselessly committed against them. At times this may have been part of systematised and brutal torture and degradation. At some point they have had to flee, pull up roots and escape to an unknown fate awaiting them in a strange and often hostile land.

Renos Papadopolous (2002) provides a working model of four phases to the refugee experience:

- Anticipation
- Devastating events
- Survival
- Adjustment.

His emphasis is on the recognition that not all refugees are traumatised. Indeed, some are truly remarkable as a testament to human resilience and endurance. Of course, what is common to all refugees is the loss of home. Home is necessary for a sense of constancy and stability; it provides a space for intimate relationships and contributes to a view of life as essentially reliable. Home grounds and provides coherence to the story of families. This loss, Papadopolous suggests, leads to a state of nostalgic yearning: 'The absence of home creates a gap in refugees which makes them feel uncontained and they then look around to fill the gap, to make up for the loss, to recreate the protective and containing membrane of home.'

For many different reasons a refugee may become known to the social worker. Their experience may encompass all that Papadopolous's phases imply and much more. They may well have very real and practical problems that require attention – housing, medical care, work, a living wage to name a few. Often the initial presentation to services pre-dates the granting of asylum status and the individual also struggles with the intricate workings of the Home Office.

It is only in this broader context of viewing the refugee experience that allows us to then make use of our understanding of trauma in this specialised area. Holding in mind the context in which these devastating events have been experienced and the consequences of this is vital in maintaining an appropriate therapeutic stance. Whilst not all refugees are traumatised, many of those who engage with services have experienced significant trauma. Making use of a psychoanalytic understanding of the impact of trauma allows a deeper understanding of the refugee's experiences and the impact this may have on the work required within social care.

I will use a psychoanalytic understanding of the impact of trauma to describe how staff are almost inevitably pulled into particular kinds of actions, repetitions of the traumatic experiences that are revived at an unconscious level. If one is alert to this in the work, it may be possible to prevent situations where, although help is available, it cannot be helpfully used; instead it becomes a kind of enclave or excursion where nothing changes. In the worst-case scenario, time, effort and money are diverted into endless cycles of unconscious repetition of the traumatic experience between patient and staff.

From a psychoanalytic perspective, trauma is thought to pierce the protective shield around the mind so that it is flooded with an excess of external stimulation. Internally there is a powerful re-activation of primitive anxieties that further overwhelm the individual. Helplessness, chaos and horror contribute to the sense that one's worst nightmares have been realised. Trauma attacks the capacity to symbolise so that thought is no longer possible, at least in the area of the trauma itself. There is inevitably a push to action and one form this may take is through the power of the Repetition Compulsion. Traumatised patients may unconsciously construct a theatre in which the traumatic scenario is endlessly repeated with the different roles of victim, perpetrator, witness and rescuer offered to others who may be drawn in. Staff will find themselves repeatedly and unconsciously drawn into re-enactments of the traumatic scenario in its various forms.

PTSD diagnoses may result from natural and man-made disasters, violence including sexual violence, incarceration and torture, and other events where extreme terror, helplessness or threat to life was experienced. The diagnosis of

Post-Traumatic Stress Disorder (PTSD) has been in common usage since the mid 1980s, originally coined in response to the experiences of Vietnam veterans in the United States. The symptoms of PTSD include nightmares, flashbacks, intrusive thoughts and images, intense physiological distress, avoidance and numbing, hyper-arousal, hyper-vigilance and exaggerated startle response.

Judith Herman (1992), an American psychiatrist, described a particular group of trauma survivors as having a condition she called complex trauma. This group included veterans, victims of domestic violence and adults who had been sexually abused as children. She felt the link with these groups was the experience of captivity, and the result was a constellation of symptoms. These included the classic PTSD features alongside dissociation, somatisation, re-victimisation, identity disturbance and affect dysregulation. This diagnosis is not yet in any formal psychiatric classificatory system but it is increasingly recognised by clinicians as a helpful description of patients who have suffered repeated, sustained or chronic traumatisation. Complex trauma presentations are common in the asylum seeker and refugee populations. Social workers will inevitably find themselves faced with difficult and at times overwhelming emotional responses to their clients. A psychoanalytic understanding of trauma can help one to understand the impact of this work on staff and provide a space in which thought may help to intervene in the inevitable push towards action.

Although the case examples I am giving are from my work as a therapist within a specialist trauma service, I believe they also have resonance across many different settings, including social work.

Mr A came to the UK as an unaccompanied minor after losing all his family in his war-torn homeland. He was clearly a survivor, someone who had found capacities inside that allowed him to keep going. When I met him, he had been in the country for four years and in that time he had been granted status and had successfully applied for British citizenship. He had learnt English and had begun a college course. What was occupying his mind at this time was his battle to obtain council housing. He had been made homeless after breaking his arm and losing his temporary job. He now lived in a hostel and was desperate to obtain a place of his own.

The battle with the council over the appropriate banding of his housing needed became the central preoccupation for the next two years. Over this time I saw Mr A on a fortnightly basis and would write supportive letters when this seemed necessary. He rarely spoke of anything to do with his life prior to arriving in the UK, and I had little sense of what had happened to him until his arrival in London. Most of our time he was focused on the council and the fight he faced. When Mr A obtained his council flat, my sense was that something inside of him collapsed. He moved into an empty, almost uninhabitable flat and broke down.

This description of the fight followed by the collapse when the aim is reached is not uncommon. As long as there is a clear fight to be won, almost unlimited internal strength might be found. The battle serves a number of purposes. Firstly it keeps one busy so that the mourning that is required for the many losses the traumatised patient faces can, for a time, be warded off. Secondly it allows the management of anxieties through defence processes such as splitting and projective identification. There is also, of course, the reality that these are battles that need to be fought in many circumstances.

In the Tavistock Trauma Service, we make use of Melanie Klein's (1946) description of the early infantile state of mind to understand the nature of the anxieties the traumatised patient faces and the defences at their disposal. Thus, the trauma results in a reactivation of powerful, infantile anxieties from the paranoid–schizoid position of early infantile life. The patient is overwhelmed by terror and dread, anxieties of disintegration and death predominate. Terrible frightening forces dominate one and there is no sense of protection or trust in the goodness of the world. The worst of infantile and childhood fears are realised.

In the normal course of development, the way an infant attempts to manage unbearable anxieties such as annihilation and disintegration is to split their feelings and experiences into categories of very good and very bad. In this way they can feel more manageable and it is only slowly as the mind develops that it can begin to integrate its view of the world. The other defence mechanism that holds sway in these early times is projective identification. What this essentially means is that what is unbearable is split off and evacuated into the mind of another. This has an impact on the other.

In time it may be possible to bring together these categories of very good and very bad in a way that allows for recognition of the way they are being attributed to individuals who are experienced as gratifying the patient's needs, or frustrating them. This opens the possibility of more mature states of mind, involving ambivalence, mourning for what has been lost and the recognition of one's own aggression. This brings guilt and the potential for reparation in what Melanie Klein (1940) described as the depressive position. We would see this gradual shift as a time in which development and change is possible but at the cost of considerable psychic pain.

For Mr A the fight with the council set up a very potent split where the council became the bad guys and I was the good guy. In work with asylum seekers, one may often see this kind of splitting with the resulting idealisation and denigration with the Home Office. The split allowed Mr A to manage his anxieties and he kept at bay the unbearable feelings he had in relation to his experiences. When he no longer had this split available, everything flooded back.

My experience with Mr A was to feel invited into being the rescuer. I would protect him from the terrible housing department who were persecuting him. Of course one of the dangers of being idealised whilst another is denigrated is that these positions can easily switch and this often meant I was anxious and uncertain. In addition, my impression was that Mr A was, at times, being aggressive and threatening to the housing staff, giving them an experience of helplessness and fear. His experiences of such profound trauma at a young age were literally unthinkable and hence he acted them out in his battles to find himself a home. One also imagines that finally winning the battle for a home also overwhelmed him with guilt for being the sole survivor of his family and gaining what they had all lost.

Massive psychic trauma collapses the distinction between the external world and internal experience: there is no longer an outside from which a perception comes or an inside which can register it. When the external world becomes a direct reflection of our worst nightmares, and our most terrifying thoughts, feelings and fantasies, then reality testing is irrelevant and the survivor enters the world of psychic equivalence. Fonagy and Target (1996) used this term to describe how mental contents can appear to correspond to physical realities. However in trauma this is reversed – it is not that perception has been contaminated by unconscious fantasies but rather that the psyche is overwhelmed by external horrors that find their equivalents in the unconscious. Our worst nightmares are realised, thought and actuality have become one. Reflection is foreclosed and thinking and perception are replaced by concrete mental entities that cannot be explored. Wilfred Bion (1959), in describing his own experiences in the trenches, emphasised how effective destroying links between thoughts can be during the trauma itself. Destroying links between thoughts allows one to fend off annihilation anxiety that is proving literally unthinkable.

This has interesting connections with neuropsychological research in trauma that demonstrates the brain's failure to formulate thoughts efficiently under extreme stress. As Van der Kolk (2014) describes, a traumatic event does not get processed in symbolic/linguistic forms as most memories are: instead it tends to be organised on a sensori-motor level – as horrific images, visceral sensations or flight/fight reactions. Storage on a sensori-motor level and not in words is supposed to explain why this type of material does not undergo the usual transforming process into autobiographical narrative memory. This leads to his oft-repeated phrase that in trauma, 'the body knows the score'.

The increased secretion of adrenaline in trauma disrupts the hippocampus, short-circuiting the system so that memories become stored as somatic sensations and visual images in the amygdala. The higher cortical structures for linguistic memory are bypassed. Fragmented sensory, affective and motor memories bombard the survivor, often seemingly without triggers. This bombardment, coupled with the sense of being unable or unwilling to find the thoughts that might attach to them, leads survivors to be increasingly withdrawn and reactive. One can also see how this connects with presentations of medically unexplained symptoms – somatisation – a common feature in complex trauma patients.

Ms C suffered significant injuries when she was the victim of a suicide bomber in a United Nations building in her Middle Eastern homeland. She was a Christian who was brought to the UK for medical treatment, and who subsequently applied for asylum. In the midst of all this, one of her brothers was kidnapped and tortured. When I met her she spoke of her hatred of this country and her mistreatment here. She was often disturbingly racist and attacking of Arab people and felt threatened by Muslims. When Ms C spoke of the English with hatred and disdain or the Home Office and its treatment of her, I would find myself thinking 'well thank goodness I am Australian, so she can't mean me'.

My sense is that she was desperately trying to find a way to keep safe in her mind her original home, and this required splitting off anything dangerous or bad into others who were different. Fakhry Davids (2011) writes of this in his paper on the 'Internal Racist', the capacity in us all to lodge what is unacceptable into the other, who is recognised as not like us. I believe my sidestepping this process in my thoughts of my own identity was an attempt to avoid the painful reality of what she was attempting to manage, which included her own aggression and fury with the English, who made her feel so vulnerable, needy and dependant. It is often true that these feelings of dependency are heightened by the system of asylum where one is unable to work, often dependent on the charity of others, and passively required to await outcomes of proceedings that may take many years.

Working with Ms C was often a very painful and difficult experience. She would speak very rapidly and in a loud, shrill voice that would feel at times as though it was reverberating inside my mind, leaving me with a headache. It is interesting to note that her major symptom after the bomb was severe headaches. When she would utter racist comments in this manner, it was often difficult to feel that I could think sufficiently to address this in a robust way. I would find instead that I was left uncomfortable with having somehow gone along with her racism. The experience for me in the room was to repeatedly find myself anxious, guilty and unable to think.

Ms C was communicating something disturbing, which she found unbearable, through projective identification. Trying to bear this, without action or attempts to rid myself of the pain and acute discomfort, was essential for beginning to offer Ms C an emotional experience which, psychoanalytically, Wilfred Bion (1959) conceptualised as containment. Bion described this notion in terms of the experience mothers offer their babies. In the normal course of development, a baby, filled with the kinds of early anxieties I described earlier, communicates this distress emotionally. It is the mother's role to try to take this in, to think about it and attempt to understand what might be going on in the baby's mind so that she might relieve this distress. Over time, with repeated experiences of containment, the baby builds up a reliable experience that someone can bear what they feel is unbearable, and thus can lessen the need to rid oneself of distress, and instead find their own ways to think about such experiences.

Ms C had every reason to feel herself in the grip of terror, dread, annhililatory and persecutory anxiety. She was trying to manage by splitting her experiences and her feelings so the new country became the bad guy and the old held everything good. She attempted to rid herself of what was unbearable through her racism. Her communication with me was a powerful experience where I was being asked to contain some of feelings she could not bear. The containment in this way is also something that I feel is part of providing a home – hopefully a temporary one – for what cannot yet be borne. In time Ms C has slowly been able to move more towards her ambivalence for both countries and has no longer spoken of racist feelings. It has been possible to mourn some of what she has lost and to feel more curious about her new country.

Discussion

In these brief vignettes I hope I have given some sense of the struggles that may face professionals in working with traumatised individuals. I have described my own experiences in a specialist trauma service but I believe they are applicable across a broad range of settings and modalities of therapy. In every relationship between a professional and an individual suffering the aftermath of trauma, there are these possibilities of enactments, of repetitions of the original traumatic scenario.

As a therapist, my own countertransference experiences can feel unbearable, and there is at times the wish to turn away. At other times I feel the pull to be active, to become caught up in the political and social realities of the patient's experience, and there can be a real threat of becoming the rescuer, and turning a blind eye to the resilience and capacities of my patients. Acknowledging the extent of human aggression and destructiveness that is part of the response to traumatic events is vital when one can be unconsciously drawn into the role of aggressor or perpetrator. Careful monitoring of the countertransference experiences, often requiring support of a team or supervision, allows for the recognition of the complexity of these encounters. Ultimately it may offer the possibility of action making way for thought, remembering rather than repetition.

Editors' afterword

Psychotherapists working with refugees have a lot in common with social workers. Not only do we also work with refugees and asylum seekers, but we risk getting caught up with enacting the same dynamics. Refugees are not the only traumatised people social workers work with. The example which springs to mind is children and adolescents who have been sexually abused within their own families. Not only is the sexual act traumatic, but it involves a parent being out of control. Very often the other parent is aware of it, but does not protect the child. As Joanne makes it clear, working with the victim may involve the breakdown of good and bad people. Where the abuser is the father, the mother is often complicit. A seven-year-old girl was sexually abused by her father for six months while her mother watched the television in the next room. When she plucked up the courage to tell her mother, she was told not to tell anyone else. She never spoke of it again until she was an adult in psychotherapy.

However, more tricky for the social worker to deal with is when the victim is involved in a repetition compulsion, where she puts herself in the way of abuse. This is not uncommon in foster placements. When MB was a newly qualified social worker she was asked to see a sixteen-year-old girl, Ella, who had some learning difficulties. She did not go out except to school and spent all her time with her father, while her mother was at work. It was suspected that there was a sexual relationship between father and daughter. Over the next few weeks Ella smartened up her appearance and even washed her hair. When MB complimented her on the improvement she became very angry and told MB she should not be a social worker. MB was left feeling very guilty and puzzled. With hindsight, Ella thought MB was sexually interested in her, projecting her own sexuality into a work relationship. Ella also projected the guilt she felt for leaving her mother out of the relationship with her father.

These sorts of enactments can be far more subtle than this and one can be in the middle of something before becoming aware of it. Supervision is essential to deal with this. The risk is that the social worker can be left with a painful countertransference experience.

Acknowledgements

I would like to thank the members of the Tavistock Trauma Service for the solid containment of working together over many years.

References

Bion, W.R. (1959) Attacks on linking. *International Journal of Psychoanalysis* 40. Reprinted in: (1967) *Second Thoughts*. London: Heinemann.

Fakhry Davids, M. (2011) *Internal Racism: A Psychoanalytic Approach to Race and Difference*. London: Palgrave Psychotherapy Series.

Fonagy, P. and Target, M. (1996). Playing with reality: 1. Theory of mind and the normal development of psychic reality. *International Journal of Psychoanalysis* 77, 217–233.

Herman, J. (1992) *Trauma and Recovery: From Domestic Violence to Political Terror*. London: Pandora.

Klein, M. (1940) Mourning and its relation to manic-depressive states. *International Journal of Psychoanalysis* 21, 125–153.

Klein, M. (1946) Notes on some schizoid mechanisms. *International Journal of Psychoanalysis* 27, 99–110.

Papadopoulos, R. (ed.) (2002) *Therapeutic Care for Refugees*. London: Karnac.

Van der Kolk, B. (2014) *The Body Keeps the Score: Mind, Brain and Body in the Transformation of Trauma*. London: Allen Lane.

PART III
Teaching

14

OBSERVATION AS A WAY OF LEARNING

Marion Bower

One of the most striking aspects of serious child abuse cases is that the abused child is not 'seen' by the various professionals who come into contact with him or her. Social workers usually come in for the most criticism, even though this blindness seems to affect all who come into contact with the child. I would like to describe a case of this sort and to put forward a suggestion of the mechanism of this blindness. The second part of this chapter looks at how the capacity for seeing in emotionally charged situations can be increased by practice and theory. The theory serves as a helpful partner for the observer.

Broken and twisted

This was a case described by a very experienced social worker to a work discussion group on a post-qualifying course. Mr and Mrs A were a comfortably-off white middle-class couple who had a ten-month-old daughter Mary. Mrs A decided to go back to work on a part-time basis, leaving Mary with her aunt who was a child minder. Mary was already known to her GP as Mrs A took her to see him frequently with minor or even imaginary ailments. When Mrs A brought Mary three times in one week, the GP decided to conduct a more careful examination. He found a lump on Mary's head and decided to send her for X-rays. It was discovered that Mary had eight partially healed fractures on various parts of her body. What was particularly horrific was that the paediatrician said that some of the fractures could only have been caused by active twisting. All the adults in the case denied causing the injuries and accusations flew backwards and forwards between them. Interestingly the GP seemed untroubled by guilt, despite missing the previous injuries. We decided to continue discussions of the case the following week.

What seemed curious was that Mary did not show any signs of pain. The social worker said that Mary always smiled at her, but the expression in her eyes was one of terror. As she said this the social worker began to shake uncontrollably, as if she was suddenly in touch with her own feelings about the case. She then remembered that Mary's aunt was no longer registered as a child minder because of cruelty to children in her care. We also wondered why neither parent had noticed Mary's pain. It seems to me now that Mary's only way of dealing with the pain of her injuries was by *dissociation*. This dissociation mirrors the apparent lack of awareness in the parents and aunt. Mrs A's frequent visits to the GP suggest she was aware that there was something wrong, but she seemed unconnected from what she knew. I think the frequent 'failure to see the child' in horrific child protection cases involves a projection of a dissociated state into the professionals. In this case the social worker's experience and sensitivity cut through this.

What is not generally realised is that 'seeing the child' has an emotional as well as visual component. It can also be developed by training and practice. The rest of this chapter describes my experience of setting up and running (with colleagues) a young child observation seminar on a post-qualifying course for childcare social workers. The course was a large one, 70 to 80 social workers who came in on two parallel days. We used an adaptation of the Tavistock Method. This was developed by a child psychotherapist called Esther Bick as a training for child psychotherapists. Students were asked to observe a child or baby in a fly-on-the-wall approach. They were to take no notes, but write up what they had observed afterwards. They were encouraged to write what they *felt* as well as what they saw. They were asked *not* to observe a child known to social services. The observations were for one hour once a week for ten weeks. Most of the students chose to observe in day nurseries, although a few people observed very young children with their mothers or carers. Parental consent was obtained for all the observations. Students took it in turn to discuss their observation in seminar groups run by leaders experienced in this type of observation. At first students were afraid they would not remember anything, but very quickly found that their capacity to remember details greatly increased. Some people were uneasy about 'doing nothing' when the adults were all busy. In fact a quiet and receptive adult was a magnet for small children, and the observers found themselves reading with children or giving a cuddle.

One of the first things to emerge in the seminar groups were observations of how little attention many of the children got in nurseries. A child could easily go for an hour without speaking to an adult. Staff tended to congregate around the kitchens. Children varied in how they coped with this. One white boy spent a long time pulling a wet cloth between his fingers. In fact a number of children were engaged in masturbatory activity as a response to loneliness. Some children had other tactics. One Afro-Caribbean boy caught the eye of members of staff and smiled at them. Usually they smiled back. While he did this he was building a house out of tiny bits of plasticine. He was building attention out of scraps. This response was very different to those children who retreated into masturbatory play. He was making the best of what was available. In social work we often have to evaluate whether or not a child is resilient. This little boy certainly was. One of the most upsetting observations was an Indian boy in a playgroup. The playgroup was 'educational'. Toys were arranged by category on tables and children were moved rapidly from table to table. The little boy sat on the floor and did not speak. The observer, who was also Indian, squatted down and talked to him. He immediately talked to her and even smiled. We thought that an observer like his mother was the reason for this. However the observer told us that one of the playgroup helpers who also spoke to him got the same response and she was white. Of course some nurseries and playgroups were excellent, but they were by no means in the majority. It raises questions about policies which depend on children being placed in nurseries from an early age. The Indian observer above commented that the playgroup was 'hostile to attachment'. This may be an issue in our society.

Observation as a developmental tool

Each group in the observation seminars had in it seven or eight members, and one seminar leader who remained a constant. This allowed the students to get to know seven or eight small children and their personalities; they also got to know each other. Learning in a small group like this is very important. It makes students aware of the importance of continuity. If one student was away for any reason, we really felt it. This attachment to an individual social worker has been eroded in recent years. 'Hot desking' breaks up friendship groups, and social workers are not encouraged to offer regular appointments to clients.

In a low-key way the seminar groups had therapeutic value. We discussed the emotional development of the children, and the students' responses to them. The focus on small children puts students in touch with younger aspects of themselves. Many of the social workers had very little teaching on their original training about physical and emotional aspects of young child development. Those students who had children of their own had an advantage. However everyone made a distinction between their own or friends' children and 'clients' children'. What they hoped or expected for clients' children was much less than for children they knew. When educational outcomes are so appalling for children in the care system this is not an academic matter.

Close contact with small children made certain aspects of the course more relevant. Freud's theory of child sexuality was accepted more readily when students saw children engaged in masturbation and sexual play. Quite often there is a resistance in recognising this in case children are blamed for sexual abuse. Students were able to observe the interaction between the child's internal world, and the external world of the nursery or other environment. The internal world is made up of objects (people) from the external world coloured by the child's feelings about them. For example, we thought that the little boy who made a house out of scraps of plasticine probably had strong, helpful internal objects. This is relevant when we have to think of the needs of children in troubled families. Some children may have a more resilient internal world than others.

John

About halfway through the ten weeks we showed the Robertsons' film *John*. This film, made in 1967, follows a 17-month-old boy who spends ten days in a residential nursery while his mother is having another baby. The nursery is part of a training institution where its young staff were on a shift system which offers fragmented care to a large group of very young children. We see John's attempts to emotionally engage with a consistent member of staff, but this is constantly disrupted. He descends into a sort of depressive breakdown. This is an immensely distressing film to watch and many people get angry with the Robertsons or the nursery. The social workers were sympathetic but viewed the film professionally. They questioned why John, with his seventeen months of 'good' care, collapses. Why does Martin, who spent eleven months in foster care, continue to fight for attention? The Robertsons' simplistic attachment theory does not explain this. One social worker commented: 'the most worrying children are the ones we hardly see'. This is the noisy gang of permanent residents who have given up having their needs met and spend most of their time shrieking, laughing and fighting, in a permanent state of manic excitement. From a psychoanalytic view this 'gang' is like those described by Herbert Rosenfeld (1971) where vulnerable aspects of the self are 'looked after' by omnipotent aspects of the self and prevented from reaching real help. John seems to have lost his good internal object and retreats into minor illness and depression. Martin, the little boy who fights for attention, has a good internal figure whom he constantly seeks to find in the external world.

Before the end of the course some students were able to apply the ideas in their workplaces, even when the workplace was not supportive. One social worker described an incident while she was on duty in a busy child protection team. She was asked to take a child who had disclosed physical abuse in school to a doctor's appointment. As she raced out of the office carrying the file she realised she had not even registered the name of the child. Remembering Bion's concept of containment she tried to think about the anxieties the child might be feeling. Then she made some time while they both sat in the car to talk about these. The little girl had an experience of a sympathetic adult, and went quite readily to the doctor. Whether a client moves on to another professional or service often depends on the quality of their first contact with a social worker. Very often a social worker looks round for a service for a child or a young person and finds that they are 'it'.

Some learning outcomes

Isabel Menzies Lyth, a psychoanalyst famous for her work in institutions caring for the vulnerable, the sick, and the very young, says:

> It's money for old rope to make people more sensitive, actually, because they want to be anyway. But when you sent them back to where they came from, and they're back in the old situation, it does not allow them to deploy more sensitivity. All that happens is that they slip back or get very disgruntled or discontented and they leave.

(Menzies Lyth, 1988)

Actually I think social workers changing jobs for a better one is quite a good out-come. A number of students got new and better jobs after the course ended. (This was not just the effect of the observation seminars but the course as a whole.) This is better than languishing in a sado-masochistic relationship with an unsatisfactory job. There will always be unsatisfactory job situations. What matters is that social workers have the confidence of their own understanding and perspective. Part of this confidence also came from the psychoanalytic theory they learned from separate lectures given by myself and other colleagues.

Observation courses

A ten-week-course like this could be either a stand-alone course or added to a qualifying or post-qualifying course. The seminar leaders would need to be familiar with the Tavistock model. It would also need to be accompanied by a theoretical module teaching basic psychoanalytic concepts, particularly those of Freud and Klein. These courses have a value in sensitising social workers to what they are observing, and observations could be made of other groups of people, such as patients on a psychiatric ward, although the issue of permission would need careful thought.

References

Menzies Lyth, I.E.P. (1988) *Containing Anxiety in Institutions*. Vols 1 and 2. London: Free Association Books.

Rosenfeld, H. (1971) A clinical aproach to the psychoanalytic theory of the life and death instincts. *International Journal of Psychoanalysis* 52, 169–178.

15

PSYCHOANALYSIS AND THE PSYCHOTHERAPIES

Institutional cleansing

Narendra Keval

Psychoanalysis is no stranger to ethnic hatred, having been marginalised by the anti-Semitism of the Viennese, non-Jewish establishments which influenced the medical and other scientific faculties of European universities. Its unpalatable ideas about the human condition were misperceived as a reflection of Jewish temperament as a race. The holocaust that eventually unfolded in the 'ethnic cleansing' and genocide of the Jews in Europe led many analysts, including Freud, to become displaced refugees. Could it be that these deeply traumatic events surface as symptoms in the way the ethnic other is treated in the body of psychoanalysis, echoing Freud's (1914) discovery that what is not remembered and worked-through is likely to be repeated?

Instead of the inner experience of the ethnic other being contained, it risks becoming marginalised and thwarted within a body of knowledge and a practice which should, one might say, know better. In this way it is given only refugee status, without a home or a receptive container that accommodates and speaks to experience across ethnicities. Having been a historical object of denigration and segregation, might this failure of understanding of the ethnic other within its own domain be a repetition of an unconscious cleansing of the subject matter?

One way to approach this negation is to locate it within a wider framework of understanding societal and organisational defences against anxiety (Menzies Lyth, 1959). Psychoanalysis and the allied disciplines, the psychotherapies, can become caught up, like any other field of inquiry and practice, in unconscious enactments that turn a blind eye to diversity and difference in society, which gets mirrored internally in its own workings. The visible portrayal of this, institutionally, is in the way various ethnic groups, particularly black people, tend to be a relative minority if not absent as patients or as professionals in this field (Fernando, 1988). Whilst this picture may be changing, racism's remarkable capacity to co-exist with support for ethnic and cultural diversity points to the difficulties in engaging with a psychic and social phenomenon that is cunning in nature, making it difficult to identify its workings objectively, but more noticeable if you are its victim.

Race: the institutional dustbin

In a work discussion-group looking at issues of race and culture as they emerge in clinical work, I was preoccupied with the geographical positioning of our seminar room in the building. We were in the last room of the corridor at the end of the building, such that if we walked any further we would have been on our way out of the building. Perhaps this location of our space for thinking said something about where race and culture as a lived experience and subject matter was being situated unconsciously in the mind of the organisation. It was placed inside the building but on the margins, edging towards the border of being 'expelled'. This is significant because it mirrors some of the struggles in the subject matter, namely who or what is given significant physical and mental space between the mainstream and its margins. The relationship says something important about how a subject matter and its peoples are being treated, whether in the minds of individuals, groups, organisations or society. It is often in these silent or subtle ways that an assault takes place in racism, which marginalises others as inadequate or inferior.

A second observation involves an organisation in which few if any of the professional therapists were from an ethnic background other than white. Members of staff from black and other minority ethnic communities were mostly personnel who were located on the relatively junior rungs of the administrative ladder, such as reception or secretarial staff. What struck me was how common it was to see a person with a black skin colour carrying a dustpan and brush. I felt there was something compelling about this observation, since it reflected a stratification inside the organisation taking place along ethnic lines, with seniority located and associated with white staff. Black skin was associated with a junior status, and with the dustpan and brush, which raised questions about the psychic and social function of this phenomenon.

Kovel's (1984) analysis of white racism suggests that the crude, violent racism of the past that characterised the colonial mentality has become transformed into a type of violence that now operates through complex market and bureaucratic forces. The brushing aside of diverse human experiences to the margins serves both a market and a psychic economy, managing anxieties that diversity and differences stir up in the psyche and society. Powerful projective mechanisms can function to stratify and marginalise people in increasingly subtle and complex forms to keep oppressive social and economic arrangements in place. This can take place across all ethnicities, not just along the black/white cleavage of power that racism has historically monopolised.

My image of the dustpan and brush may be telling. The unconscious denigration of black skin is reproduced socio-economically by marginalising, expelling or cleansing-out blacks. In this way, their inner experience is brushed into the dustbin of our ethnically stratified society, through projective mechanisms that psychically and economically lock particular ethnicities (blacks in particular) into oppressive arrangements. These arrangements are likely to play out in ever more complex ways as our society becomes an increasingly global village with complicated migratory movements and journeys across borders. According to this view, new ethnicities and cleavages of power relations will become recruited into a historical drama that institutionalises racism. This suggests that it is not only our infantile past that we are compelled to repeat but also our historical race relations at the group and societal level.

For those caught up in it, the emotional ramifications of institutionalised forms of racism are profoundly disturbing. Those on the receiving end not only fail to be properly heard and understood but feel caught up in a racist perception or gaze that does not belong to them. As I explored in an earlier chapter, this thwarts the capacity to exercise one's emotional freedom. To withhold true recognition can amount to a psychic murder, which is always present, to one degree or another, in racist attitudes that marginalise, devalue or degrade. The subjective experience of feeling invisible or marginal is not something that has been looked at in much detail, but these conversations frequently happen behind closed doors between people of minority communities who often report a pervasive and painful feeling of being excluded or deemed invisible in a group of predominantly white people. Whether the same experience is replicated with different ethnicities is an interesting question, but it is an unconscious process that can be painfully bewildering for those on the receiving end.

Vignette 1

A colleague, the only black person amongst a white staff of clinicians, voiced her concern about the lack of space to think about black people and their experience of racism. The response from a white colleague trying to place this on the agenda for a meeting was that some of these clinicians did not want to be thinking about all this 'race stuff', they just want to get on with the work. There was an interesting silence when a question was asked as to what that meant – 'to be getting on with the work'.

Such a comment reflects an artificial split in which the 'race stuff' is marginalised in relation to the 'real' and central work of therapy. The assumption in this group was that the real work constituted depth and complexity, whilst issues of race are externally located and operate at the surface like skin, somewhat superficial in nature.

Here, one can see how quickly the structure of her thinking started to mirror the structure of how racism operates. First, to create an artificial split between the real and the superficial 'race stuff', then projection across this divide of what is deemed to be of less value or worthy of consideration. Race is then 'stuffed' (projected) with fantasies and feelings that are conveniently evacuated and dis-owned so that both the subject matter and the black colleague, by implication, are unwittingly marginalised. This is an experience that black people often consciously and unconsciously register, which leaves a feeling of being unheard or invisible.

At a small-group level, the paralysing influence of this process can sometimes be ameliorated by attempting to recognise that there is an unconscious malignant process at play even when it is difficult to name it and one cannot be sure what is going on. The recognition that there is a problem re-engages the feeling of emotional vitality that becomes temporarily attacked and paralysed by a group process which, while not overtly racist, can instigate an insidious process of marginalisation on the basis of ethnic difference.

Training and supervision

Some of the understandable challenges and conundrums of engaging with this complex psychic and social problem are often met with a stance of political correctness that can unfortunately create more difficulties than it resolves. For example, current training curricula risk mirroring racist dynamics by tagging on issues of ethnicity, race or racism in a rather concrete way. It is not unlike creating ethnic ghettos in society, which are apt to provide psychic pathways for racism. Attempts to speak to the subject matter sometimes end up as an area of applied work – an anthropological specimen that runs the risk of doing more to extend the conceptual boundaries of a theory than integrate the subjective experience of the ethnic other into its own theorising. This is a thorny issue that cannot be easily resolved, since it is a matter of debate when a body of theory and practice is being used to illuminate and understand the phenomenon under study or 'colonise' it, repeating the very dynamics of racism in its desire to validate itself as 'open' and 'responsive' to these issues.

The understandable focus on the inner world of the patient within the consulting room can sometimes get caught up with a view that sees the external world as a potential source of contamination by psychosocial processes, such as racism. It is not too difficult to see that this can potentially re-create some of the very dynamics that underpin the structure of racist thought and feeling – the desire to regress to a dyadic space at the cost of a capacity to develop triangularity, which forces a recognition of the complexities of life and living. Perhaps as a defence against the difficulties of thinking creatively about difference and diversity one can witness attitudes of polite indifference, ignorance and sometimes arrogance that veil anxieties to do with bewilderment, uncertainty and fear.

Psychic life does not operate independently of the way our society has evolved along stratified lines to bolster unequal power relationships between ethnicities. In both its malignant and benign forms, racial or ethnic myths and pressures have a profound effect on one's conscious and unconscious attitudes to the developmental tasks that have to be negotiated on the path towards emotional maturity. One of the clinical challenges is to understand the inner world in the context of early life experiences and relationships situated in the ambience of the ethnic or cultural milieu, creating a mosaic of meanings to be understood in the clinical encounter.

Transference, rightly deemed the pinnacle of working analytically, also concerns the repetition of history – not only early infantile relations but ideologies that underpin the dynamics of race relations in the here and now, re-enacted from one generation to the next. One of the most challenging tasks in our professions is to understand the complexities of how infantile and ideological pasts link up in the unconscious to give shape to all that the patient brings to the consulting room.

Vignette 2

A black trainee amongst a white group of therapists in training, whom I knew to be quite vocal, gradually began to withdraw in silence in one of my teaching seminars. I thought about how I could speak to this observation without being presumptuous and intrusive. I eventually decided to speak to her directly in a separate meeting because of my concern that it might affect her learning through her lack of engagement. I simply stated my observation to her.

She said she was relieved that I had brought it up as it was something she had noticed in herself in the seminar but did not understand what was happening to her nor how she could speak about it. She had observed the same thing happening in other situations with the same group of fellow students, with whom she got on well. When I asked about her experience of the content of the seminar and discussion she was able to elaborate on how she had been feeling increasingly different and isolated as a black person on the course, particularly when she felt much of the theoretical and clinical work did not speak to her experience as a black woman with her own culture and customs. Instead of vocalising her views she withdrew and re-directed her anger and protest by moving her emotional experience to the margins and shutting herself off.

Aside from whatever else was going on that I was not privy to, the striking thing to witness was the change in her demeanour following our brief conversation. In subsequent seminars she was more lively and willing to debate and participate, which suggests that she had managed to recover her potency that had become temporarily paralysed in the group. This is a crucial point in the black experience of racism, where there is an overwhelming sense of feeling powerless to speak to an experience that is difficult to name and pinpoint. There have been many anecdotal reports of this paralysing silence, which needs to be further investigated.

It is possible that a shared unconscious fantasy may be at play in these situations, ascribing dominant and submissive roles and voices according to racial/cultural categories. This shared fantasy may be taken up and used in ways that are peculiar to the individuals and groups concerned, and is not unlike how couples might function in a dysfunctional marriage or partnership (Dicks, 1967).

While, consciously, I thought the thinking in the seminar was meant to be inclusive, the black trainee's experience suggested otherwise, culminating in a subtle shift of her experience towards the margins that was colluded with by her withdrawal.

Even my tentative attempts to speak to this seemed to have freed her up, enabling her to recover her voice. I think this phenomenon occurs in many organisations but the marginalisation is colluded with by all participants and is often difficult to name. Finding a voice representing the experience of those from non-white ethnic backgrounds in training curricula is particularly challenging given these subtle processes of marginalisation, but my examples also provide some hope about naming and identifying them so that possibilities for change can be thought about.

Vignette 3

The clinical supervision space can be conceptualised as a triangular space, in which the supervisor's task is to assist the trainee to develop a state of mind in which he can be receptive and reflective about his work. When a supervisor reflects on the dynamics of a therapist/patient couple to make inferences about the underlying difficulties that the patient may experience, this helps the therapist create a state of mind in which he can become receptive and reflective, open to impressions and be able to take a third position, from where he can observe himself while participating with the patient. This creation of a triangular space is crucial in the therapist's development if he is to help his patient identify with and internalise a benign thinking object. However, when difficulties arise which fail to be adequately contained in supervision, these can result in the therapist feeling too vulnerable to manage the clinical situation and lead to acting-out by both therapist and patient.

The following vignette describes a situation which was reported to me in a consultation by a male Pakistani Muslim therapist who had been the subject of racist remarks with threats of overt violence in a psychotherapy group he was running. This was initially run with a female co-therapist of Spanish descent who decided to leave the institution. After the group members were told of her decision some months prior to her departure, members expressed feelings of being rejected and not good enough for the therapist to stay and work with them.

Following her departure, the group's anger and resentment turned on the Muslim therapist with a fantasy that she left because he had become violent and got rid of her. What most of these patients had in common was an early history of being adopted, the trauma of which found fertile ground in the departure of the co-therapist. Feelings of being rejected and wounded found a convenient pathway by using the Muslim therapist's ethnicity to express their hurt and wish for revenge. The predominant feeling in the group was that they had been deserted and left in the hands of a therapist who was the culprit. When two male members turned on him by making racist remarks, the therapist noted that the rest of the group watched this attack with equanimity, perhaps seeing a reversal of what they felt had been inflicted on them by the therapist couple.

While the therapist attempted to interpret some of these feelings in the group, he realised that he was faced with a gang-type mentality which was difficult to reason with. The impasse was all the more difficult to resolve as he told me he found the racist comments had temporarily affected his capacity to think coherently, as if his thinking had been attacked as well. He also lacked his co-therapist's support in the face of this assault, and it was apparent when listening to him that he had a variety of unresolved feelings about her departure. Some of these had been explored between them and jointly in supervision, but the matter of his race as a potential vehicle that could be used destructively was not discussed at all.

While the supervisor tried to help the therapist contain the destructiveness of the group, he felt that this did not address the specific issue of how his race was being used as a weapon to express their anger, nor the difficulty of managing racist projections when these are often part and parcel of daily living for black people in the outside world.

The analytic task was clear enough. One has to be receptive to the racist projections and allow oneself the wish to retaliate, but then engage the capacity to think and explore with them: what was being communicated by their wish to wound him in this way, given the departure of the co-therapist? This task would be difficult enough, given that racist projections attack the very links in thinking that one needs to be able to do, but without the support of his co-therapist and supervisor it was made more difficult still.

In this particular case the supervisor attempted to help the therapist by asking him to obtain some reading material pertaining to race issues so that he felt better contained to manage the group. This idea was meant to provide an alternative source of support for the therapist, albeit an intellectual one, in the face of the group assault, which he was now facing without the support of his co-therapist. Unfortunately, thinking about his ethnicity was lodged outside the supervision space, leaving the therapist uncontained. In the following session, one of the male patients lost control of his anger, this time threatening to hit a female patient, as if to enact an ongoing fantasy that it was the violence perpetrated by the black therapist on his co-therapist that drove her to leave.

This was a group defence against acknowledging the profound feelings of rejection, loss and rage at having suffered a 'primal wound' (Verrier, 1993) from maternal abandonment, a dynamic now being repeated in the group. They found a way to communicate their experience of being dropped from the co-therapist's mind by finding a dramatic and volatile way of ensuring that they were seen and heard, getting under the therapist's skin by targeting his ethnicity to express their hurt and grievance. His ability to cope was, however, compromised, not only because of his unresolved feelings about his co-therapist's departure, but also because the supervision space did not keep the issue of his ethnicity in mind, to be explored and understood in the context of the group process. Instead, thinking about this was exported to an 'adoptive mother' in the form of an idea of readings on race which was expected to contain the therapist's anxiety, mirroring a dynamic in which adopted patients are often expected to embrace their adoptive mother and new home, without having processed the complex feelings of being abandoned by their biological mothers. It leaves them with a profound feeling that a vital area of their early life has not been thought about or articulated, but which continually haunts them in their future relationships (Samuel, 2003).

Professional practice

Professionals can face pressures both from within and outside their organisations to create certainties in their work which often prove to be untenable. This is sometimes expressed in a culture of prescriptive thinking or a 'manual' for thinking that aims to short-circuit the difficulty of learning from experience and a genuine labour of ideas. Prescriptive thinking often results in a purely intellectual approach taken to the subject matter, draining it of any feeling or substance so that it becomes sanitised and safe to work with. It probably accounts for the disjunction between the experience of racism and the language used to describe it, questioning to what extent it is possible to remain engaged and able to articulate an experience that arouses many volatile feelings without explaining or sanitising it away.

The splitting of thought and feeling is a symbolic violence that is often discernible in attempts to theorise or converse about the subject in professional discussions, which sometimes make them appear two-dimensional, flat or sterile. The danger is to mimic the very simplicity and lack of depth or dimensionality that form the fabric of racist structures of thought and feeling. It can give the impression of furthering our knowledge but can close off any prospect of a depth to our understanding. In short, just as the ethnic other is treated as a one-dimensional entity in racial hatred and violence, so too is there the danger that our language and thinking will be devoid of any curiosity and imagination and suffer the same fate.

The attack on meaning can be often observed in groups engaged in discussions about race or racism, with a surprising regularity of comments about the difficulty of grasping one's thoughts and the substance of thought, as if the thoughts will slip away. Comments such as 'It is difficult to articulate what I mean', 'I am not making sense', 'I cannot put it into words', 'It is not coming out correctly', 'I am talking gibberish', 'I do not know what I am saying', and so on, indicate the difficulty in creating a semantic container via the linking of words to create meaning.

Vignette 4

A black social worker was faced with a barrage of racist remarks when she visited an elderly client in her home. As her client needed to be taken into hospital for medical help, she contacted her colleagues. Upon their arrival, her white colleagues witnessed the racist abuse and refused to take the client to hospital, leaving their black colleague to attend to the client alone. They seemed to have interpreted the 'anti-racist' policy and procedures so concretely that they felt no obligation to assist their abusive client nor think about helping their black colleague to contain the situation. Their 'anti-racist' position left their black colleague alone to deal with the vulnerable and hostile client. Had the ambulance staff and social worker been able to recover a space to think and work together collaboratively they may have been able to rescue themselves from being drawn into the client's uncontrollable anxiety and aggression.

The elderly client was already highly anxious about her feelings of helplessness and dependency and when the suggestion of being taken into hospital was made this would have elevated her anxiety even further, uncertain as she was about her safety and wellbeing. These feelings found their target in the black social worker, who was already the object of racist hatred at the door, which became more severe when the client had to contemplate the prospect of placing her safety in her hands. Hospitals are anxiety-provoking places, but here the black foreigner and 'foreign experience' got equated concretely via skin colour. Had there been a space to disentangle and reduce her level of anxiety it would have enabled the client to receive the proper help she needed at the hospital despite her obnoxious behaviour.

On this occasion, the policing functions of statutory regulation made it difficult to think, and colluded with the very splitting that is characteristic of racist thinking and feeling. Instead of collaboration there was an attack on creating links that could have enabled more productive thinking to take place between them that would have contained both the client and the situation.

The study group: a space to explore race

Given the difficulties that can arise for both therapists and supervisors in thinking about race and racism in the clinical situation, the study-group format can bring anxieties about these issues to the surface in a less threatening manner, providing that they are thought about in a considered way. The task becomes one of enabling participants to use their own experience as a potential resource for grappling with difficult questions and issues about race. This involves creating a format for learning which relies less on prescriptive thinking and more on a free-associative approach that encourages them to observe and share their own thinking, feeling and behaviour.

The task is to facilitate an attitude of inquiry into the way they relate to the material at hand, as a means of understanding how the phenomenon operates. This includes observing and commenting on what emerges in their relations to each other and to the consultant in the here and now of the session. In work discussions on race or racism the polarity of thinking and feeling seems to arise as a matter of course as groups grapple with a harsh superego that emerges to 'police' impulses, revealing the limited space for thinking that results. Thinking becomes concrete so that words are felt like missiles, creating an accusatory atmosphere where the desire for absolute certainty barely disguises the arrogance in the claims to know what is the right and wrong way to think. These potentially paralysing moments of narrow-mindedness are usually located in certain individuals, based on their valency in the group which has unconsciously recruited them. The challenge then is how to avoid getting caught up in the grip of a judgemental superego so that a more fluid space can be created in which there is room for uncertainty and the exercise of curiosity, without the wish for foreclosure of meaning.

When the group is working well the atmosphere is palpably different because there is literally more space to breathe and think more imaginatively and fluidly, but the residue of depressive feelings is not to be underestimated. This is to be expected as the difficulties of truly engaging with the issues of ethnicity and race start to become more apparent (Keval, 2005).

Editors' afterword

Both of us have taught social workers over many years. So Keval's chapter had resonance for us about the importance of understanding unconscious processes in the life of a training group, and we asked him if we could include it in this volume. While it is not describing a social work training seminar, and the focus is on clinical interpretation, there is nevertheless much to learn from it for social work education. Keval's focus is primarily on the dynamics of unprocessed racism brought to the fore through the anxieties brought about by the 'not knowing' nature of learning. It speaks not only to the experiences of a black lecturer but also offers a way to think about how racial differences in a group, and racial differences between the facilitator of a group and its members, must be understood to avoid significant acting out or the depletion of learning.

Social work training has over many years been interested in promoting Anti-Discriminatory Practice, something that we are very proud of. But if these dynamics are left misunderstood or unattended to, training groups can turn from ADP to AEE – Anti-Educational Experiences.

References

Dicks, H. (1967) *Marital Tensions, Clinical Studies Towards a Psychological Theory of Interaction.* London: Karnac.

Fernando, S. (1988) *Race and Culture in Psychiatry.* Kent: Croom Helm.

Freud, S. (1914) 'Remembering, Repeating and Working-Through Further Recommendations on the Technique of Psycho-Analysis II,' (1911–1913): the case of Schreber, papers on technique and other works. *Standard Edition* 12, 145–156. London: Hogarth Press.

Keval, N. (2005) Racist states of mind. In: Bower, M. (ed.) *Psychoanalytic Theory for Social Work Practice: Thinking Under Fire.* London: Routledge, pp. 30–43.

Kovel, J. (1984) *White Racism, a Psychohistory.* New York: Columbia University Press.

Menzies-Lyth, I. (1959) The functioning of social systems as a defence against anxiety. *Human Relations* 13, 95–121.

Samuel, H. (2003) Adoption: some clinical features of adults who have been adopted and the difficulties of helping them in NHS psychotherapy. *Psychoanalytic Psychotherapy* 17(3), 206–218.

Verrier, N.N. (1993) *The Primal Wound: Understanding the Adopted Child.* Baltimore: Gateway Press.

USEFUL TEXTS

Anderson, R. (ed.) (1992) *Clinical Lectures on Klein and Bion.* London: Routledge.

Bower, M. (ed.) (2005) *Psychoanalytic Theory for Social Work Practice.* London: Routledge.

Bower, M., Hale, R. and Wood, H. (eds) (2013) *Addictive States of Mind.* London: Karnac.

Rosenfeld, H. (1971) A clinical approach to the psychoanalytic theory of the life and death instincts. In: Spillius, E. (ed.) *Melanie Klein Today.* London: Routledge.

Steiner, J. (1993) *Psychic Retreats.* London: Routledge.

Trowell, J. and Bower, M. (eds) (1995) *The Emotional Needs of Young Children and their Families.* London: Routledge.

INDEX

Page numbers in italics refer to figures.

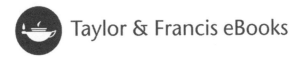

Taylor & Francis eBooks

Helping you to choose the right eBooks for your Library

Add Routledge titles to your library's digital collection today. Taylor and Francis ebooks contains over 50,000 titles in the Humanities, Social Sciences, Behavioural Sciences, Built Environment and Law.

Choose from a range of subject packages or create your own!

Benefits for you
- » Free MARC records
- » COUNTER-compliant usage statistics
- » Flexible purchase and pricing options
- » All titles DRM-free.

Benefits for your user
- » Off-site, anytime access via Athens or referring URL
- » Print or copy pages or chapters
- » Full content search
- » Bookmark, highlight and annotate text
- » Access to thousands of pages of quality research at the click of a button.

eCollections – Choose from over 30 subject eCollections, including:

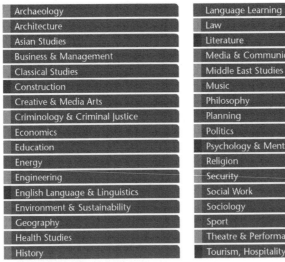

Archaeology	Language Learning
Architecture	Law
Asian Studies	Literature
Business & Management	Media & Communication
Classical Studies	Middle East Studies
Construction	Music
Creative & Media Arts	Philosophy
Criminology & Criminal Justice	Planning
Economics	Politics
Education	Psychology & Mental Health
Energy	Religion
Engineering	Security
English Language & Linguistics	Social Work
Environment & Sustainability	Sociology
Geography	Sport
Health Studies	Theatre & Performance
History	Tourism, Hospitality & Events

For more information, pricing enquiries or to order a free trial, please contact your local sales team:
www.tandfebooks.com/page/sales

Printed and bound by CPI Group (UK) Ltd, Croydon, CR0 4YY

29/10/2024

01780548-0001